# GUIDELINES
## ─── FOR ───
# CARDIAC
# REHABILITATION
# PROGRAMS

## AMERICAN ASSOCIATION
## OF CARDIOVASCULAR AND
## PULMONARY REHABILITATION

Human Kinetics Books
Champaign, Illinois

**Library of Congress Cataloging-in-Publication Data**

Guidelines for cardiac rehabilitation programs / by American
    Association of Cardiovascular and Pulmonary Rehabilitation.
            p.   cm.
        Includes bibliographical references.
        Includes index.
        ISBN 0-87322-304-7
        1. Heart--Diseases--Exercise therapy--Standards.   2. Heart-
    -Diseases--Patients--Rehabilitation--Standards.   I. American
    Association of Cardiovascular & Pulmonary Rehabilitation.
        [DNLM: 1. Heart Diseases--rehabilitation.   WG 200 G946]
    RC684.E9G84      1991
    616.1'206515--dc20
    DNLM/DLC
    for Library of Congress                                                     90-4944
                                                                                    CIP

ISBN: 0-87322-304-7

Developmental Editor:  Christine Drews
Assistant Editors:  Dawn Levy and Timothy Ryan
Copyeditor:  Wendy Nelson
Proofreader:  Linda Siegel
Indexer:  Sheila Ary
Production Director:  Ernie Noa
Typesetters:  Sandra Meier and Kathy Boudreau-Fuoss
Text Design:  Keith Blomberg
Text Layout:  Denise Lowry
Cover Design:  Jack Davis
Printer:  Braun-Brumfield

Printed in the United States of America

10   9   8   7   6   5   4   3   2   1

**Human Kinetics Books**
A Division of Human Kinetics Publishers, Inc.
Box 5076, Champaign, IL 61825-5076
1-800-747-4457

*UK Office:*
**Human Kinetics Publishers (UK) Ltd.**
PO Box 18
Rawdon, Leeds LS19 6TG
England
(0532) 504211

The initial development of these guidelines took place at a weekend meeting in Cincinnati, Ohio, when the original committee gathered for a philosophical discussion and groundwork session. Once the goals, objectives, and baseline philosophy were established, the writing became a manageable task designed to fill a void in the existing literature.

These individuals formed the original committee and were the major writers of the document as it is now presented:

Kathy Berra, BSN
Palo Alto YMCA
Palo Alto, California

Barry A. Franklin, PhD
William Beaumont Hospital
Royal Oak, Michigan

Linda K. Hall, PhD, Chairperson
Allegheny General Hospital
Pittsburgh, Pennsylvania

William Herbert, PhD
Virginia Tech
Blacksburg, Virginia

Martha Livingston, RN, MS, MBA
Central DuPage Hospital
Winfield, Illinois

Curt Meyer, MS
Lee Memorial Hospital
Fort Myers, Florida

Chip Span, MS
St. Francis Hospital
Greenville, South Carolina

Nanette K. Wenger, MD
Emory University School of Medicine
Atlanta, Georgia

Kimberly L. Wood, PhD
University of South Carolina
Aiken, South Carolina

The entire 1988 and 1989 board of directors of the AACVPR reviewed this document and provided editorial and revisionary comment. An outside panel consisting of Robert DeBusk, MD, Stanford University School of Medicine; Gerald Fletcher, MD, Emory University School of Medicine; Barbara Fletcher, MN, RN, The Emory Clinic; Paul Ribisl, PhD, Wake Forest University; and John D. Cantwell, MD, Georgia Baptist Medical Center, also served as reviewers before final editing. Final editing was accomplished by Barry A. Franklin, PhD, of William Beaumont Hospital, Royal Oak, Michigan, and Linda K. Hall, PhD, Allegheny General Hospital, Pittsburgh, Pennsylvania.

Photos on pp. 1 and 10 are printed courtesy of Palo Alto YMCA Cardiac Therapy Program, Palo Alto, CA; those on pp. 2, 6, 21, 35, and 37(bottom) are courtesy of Milwaukee County Medical Complex, Milwaukee, WI; those on pp. 9, 13, 27, 28, and 49 are courtesy of Cardio Pulmonary Rehabilitation Institute, Seattle, WA; those on pp. 11, 23, 29, 36, 39, 53, and 55 are courtesy of William Beaumont Hospital Cardiac Rehabilitation Program, Royal Oak, MI; those on pp. 33, 37(top), 43, 44, 45, 47, 48, and 50 are courtesy of Allegheny General Hospital, Pittsburgh, PA; and those on pp. 17, 30, and 40 are courtesy of Stead Health and Fitness Center, Pomona Valley Hospital Medical Center, Pomona, CA.

# Contents

**Chapter 1  Program Structure, Risk Stratification, and Monitoring Rationale**  1

Introduction  1
The Process  3
Levels of Risk Stratification  5
Continuous ECG Monitoring During Phase II Cardiac Exercise Therapy:
  Rationale and Recommendations  5
References  7

**Chapter 2  Graded Exercise Testing and Exercise Prescription**  9

Graded Exercise Testing  9
Contraindications to Exercise Testing  10
Exercise Training and Prescription  10
Contraindications to Exercise Training  12
Safety of Cardiac Exercise Therapy  12
Is High-Intensity Training Justified for Cardiac Patients?  13
References  14

**Chapter 3  Patient Assessment and Educational Programming**  17

Inpatient, Immediate Post-Hospital, Extended Outpatient, and Maintenance Cardiac
  Rehabilitation Programming  17
Educational Services  20
References  23

**Chapter 4  Program Evaluation and Efficacy Measures**  27

Assessing Program Effectiveness  27
References  31

**Chapter 5  Personnel for Cardiovascular Rehabilitation Services**  33

Competency Standards  34
Utilization of Exercise Services: Considerations Regarding Safety and Supervision  38
References  40

**Chapter 6  Guidelines for Record Keeping on Participants
          in Cardiac Rehabilitation Programs**  43

In-Hospital Rehabilitation  44
Outpatient Rehabilitation  44
Maintenance Program  45
References  46

## Chapter 7   Management of Emergencies          47

Training and Certification  48
Early Warning Signs and Symptoms of Increasing Risk  48
Interventions  49
Emergency Equipment  50
Documentation  51
References  52

## Chapter 8   Facilities and Equipment          53

In-Hospital Phase  53
Early Ambulatory Outpatient Therapeutic Program  54
Maintenance Program  55
Conclusion  56
References  56

## Appendix A   Sample Forms          59

## Appendix B   Position Paper: Scientific Evidence of the Value of Cardiac Rehabilitation Services With Emphasis on Patients Following Myocardial Infarction          75

Section 1: Exercise Conditioning Component  77
Section 2: The Efficacy of Risk Factor Intervention and Psychosocial Aspects
  of Cardiac Rehabilitation  89

Index  105
About the AACVPR  109

*Chapter 1*

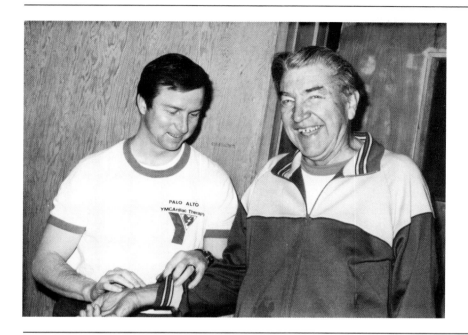

# *Program Structure, Risk Stratification, and Monitoring Rationale*

Cardiac rehabilitation was formally introduced in the 1960s on an in-patient basis as it was discovered that patients improved when they were ambulating rather than lying in bed for extended periods. Since then, the medical and surgical interventions for cardiovascular disease have changed dramatically. As a result, increasing numbers of patients are surviving cardiovascular events that formerly would have meant death. With the changing nature of interventional methodologies and with new knowledge regarding risk factors, both genetic and behavioral, it becomes necessary to redefine cardiac rehabilitation with regard to stages, risk stratification, and monitoring rationale.

**Since the 1960s, interventions for cardiovascular disease have changed dramatically, making it necessary to redefine some areas of cardiac rehabilitation.**

## Introduction

A. This report is intended as a guide for
   1. Professionals developing new cardiovascular rehabilitation programs

**The AACVPR guidelines emphasize the rehabilitative needs of the *individual* patient.**

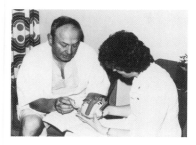

**Exercise-based cardiac rehabilitation and risk factor modification programs significantly decrease mortality.**

2. Physicians referring patients for cardiac rehabilitation services
3. Health and allied health professionals updating and/or participating in the delivery of cardiac rehabilitation services
4. Health care insurers evaluating cardiac rehabilitation programs for reimbursement
5. Educators training the aforementioned professionals
6. Patients participating in cardiac rehabilitation programs

B. The American Association of Cardiovascular and Pulmonary Rehabilitation (AACVPR) guidelines may differ in the following ways from guidelines previously published by other professional societies and voluntary health organizations:

1. An emphasis on the rehabilitative care needs of the individual patient. These needs are determined by both the primary care physician and rehabilitation staff.
2. At entry into the rehabilitative program, desired outcomes for each patient are delineated.
3. Both patient performance and rehabilitation program components are evaluated regularly. These outcome measures are based upon attainment of the goals established at the beginning of the program.
4. Rehabilitation needs are viewed with a broader scope in regard to eligibility criteria for patient participation. Previously underserved populations are addressed in the current guidelines.
5. The use of contemporary technology (home-based educational programs, flexible monitoring, risk stratification, etc.) is encouraged to provide flexibility in delivering services.
6. An increased emphasis on the educational and counseling components and incorporation of sound principles of adult learning are inherent in the current guidelines.
7. A focus on limiting the costs and increasing the accessibility to large numbers of low-risk patients. This approach, when safety is not compromised, may permit an increase in the duration and intensity of services provided to the smaller percentage of high-risk, medically complicated patients.
8. Current references and contemporary national guidelines (such as the National Cholesterol Education Program) are used to complement selected components of the *Guidelines for Cardiac Rehabilitation Programs*.

C. Background information

Prior to the early 1970s, cardiovascular rehabilitation predominantly involved patients recovering from an uncomplicated myocardial infarction, including some with concomitant angina pectoris. Typically, exercise training was initiated later and more gradually than is common currently. Only limited risk-factor modification was recommended, predominantly because the available data base gave only limited support to the view that modifying risk factors would improve patient outcome. However, two recent studies using meta-analysis have confirmed that exercise-based cardiac rehabilitation and risk factor modification programs significantly decrease mortality.[1,2]

As a general rule, patients recovering from coronary bypass surgery, coronary angioplasty, and other cardiac problems were assigned to the same care model. However, there was still suboptimal tailoring of the rehabilitative regimen to meet individual patients' needs based on their previous habits, their desired lifestyles, their behaviors that need intervention, and the severity of their diseases.

Progress in the understanding of cardiovascular disease management has recently led to changes in the role of cardiac rehabilitation to now include[3-19]

- increased cost of rehabilitation services, with a resultant alteration of the cost:benefit ratio;[19]
- information regarding the risk status of coronary patients and its application to exercise therapy;
- information about coronary risk factors and benefits of their modification; and
- information about behavioral change and the approaches for its promulgation.

A broad spectrum of patients are now considered eligible for cardiac rehabilitation services. Included are the traditional patients of past years: myocardial infarction, coronary bypass, and angioplasty patients. Additionally, coronary patients with or without residual ischemia, heart failure, and arrhythmias; a variety of categories of patients with nonischemic heart disease; patients with concomitant pulmonary disease; patients who have undergone new interventions such as pacemaker or cardioverter-defibrillator implantation, heart valve repair or replacement, and cardiac transplantation; elderly patients; and medically complex patients are now included in the cardiac rehabilitation spectrum.

There is also new technology to assist health care professionals in the delivery of cardiac rehabilitation services. This technology can provide extended ECG monitoring capabilities (for hospital-based or home training programs),[4] computerized maintenance of patient records and trends, and home-based educational programs for the patient and the family.

The approaches to implement behavioral change include the initial transmission of cognitive information, subsequent skill-building and practice, and reinforcement of the desired behavioral changes.[11] This aspect of rehabilitative care, exemplified by coronary risk reduction, typically entails a longer time than does improvement of functional capacity by exercise training.

**A broad spectrum of patients are now considered eligible for cardiac rehabilitation services.**

## The Process

### Definition

*Cardiac rehabilitation* is the process by which the person with cardiovascular disease, including but not limited to patients with coronary heart disease, is restored to and maintained at his or her optimal physiological, psychological, social, vocational, and emotional status.

### Application

Application of this process should include the perspective of individual patient needs rather than the traditional generic program. Intervention is prescribed based on three or four phases—Phase I: the hospital

**The cardiac rehabilitation process should include the perspective of individual patient needs rather than the traditional generic program.**

inpatient period (ordinarily 6 to 14 days for patients with acute myocardial infarction or following coronary artery bypass surgery); Phase II: the convalescent stage following hospital discharge (generally up to 12 weeks' duration); Phase III: the extended, supervised outpatient program (usually 4 to 6 or more months' duration); Phase IV: the ongoing maintenance period (indefinite length).

| | |
|---|---|
| **In-Hospital** (Phase I) | Rehabilitation is initiated immediately in the form of education (i.e., informal discussions with nurses and physicians) and counseling. Therapy, in the form of range-of-motion activities, intermittent sitting or standing, and walking, is then applied according to physician referral and at the level determined by the physician or staff. The purpose of this phase is, in part, to reduce the deconditioning that normally accompanies prolonged bed rest. |
| **Post-Hospital/ Immediate Exercise Intervention** (Phase II) | Exercise therapy is ordered by the physician/cardiac rehabilitation staff for low-, moderate-, or high-risk patients as determined from medical history, graded exercise test results, and documentation of arrhythmias, left ventricular function, or concurrent disease.[4] Ideally, this stage should be initiated within 3 weeks of hospital discharge. Additionally, risk-factor education and psychological and vocational needs are met as ordered, with desired outcomes specified by the physician/cardiac rehabilitation staff. |
| **Post-Hospital/ Extended Outpatient and Exercise Maintenance** (Phases III and IV) | Patients are moved into the exercise maintenance stage when stabilized cardiovascular and physiological responses to exercise have been obtained and the desired outcome from exercise therapy has been achieved or no additional progress is evident. |

**The purpose of Phase I is, in part, to reduce deconditioning caused by prolonged bed rest.**

**Ideally, Phase II should be initiated within 3 weeks of hospital discharge.**

**Phase III and IV interventions begin when responses are stable and exercise outcomes have been achieved.**

Patients may be transferred up and down through levels as the disease progresses, regresses, or appears unchanged. This document is written with the knowledge that, for many participants, clinical status will not change at hospital discharge. Certain ''high-risk'' patients will remain clinically ''high risk'' for years. These patients may be excellent candidates for supervised outpatient therapeutic programs; alternatively, logistics may dictate that they continue their rehabilitation program on their own at home. All efforts should be made to help moderate- and high-risk patients make the transition from direct medical supervision to reduced medical surveillance while maintaining maximum safety through discharge education, appropriate exercise guidelines, and sign and symptom monitoring. Independence and the adoption of self-monitoring skills should be a primary goal of all rehabilitation programs.

## Levels of Risk Stratification

The type and duration of supervision and frequency of monitoring should be guided by the level of risk (low, moderate, or high) in which the patient has been placed. The levels of risk are delineated below (Table 1.1) using data harvested from the patient's medical history, clinical course, physiological variables, and other test results, and are regarded as minimal guidelines for risk stratification;[3-13,16-18] however, categorization need not be limited to nor include every characteristic.

**Table 1.1  Guidelines for Risk Stratification**

| Risk level | Characteristics |
| --- | --- |
| Low | Uncomplicated clinical course in hospital[5] |
| | No evidence of myocardial ischemia[3,4,5,9,13] |
| | Functional capacity $\geq$ 7 METs[5] |
| | Normal left ventricular function (EF > 50%)[3,4,5] |
| | Absence of significant ventricular ectopy[18] |
| Intermediate (Moderate) | ST-segment depression $\geq$ 2 mm flat or downsloping[3,4,5,9,12] |
| | Reversible thallium defects[3,7] |
| | Moderate to good left ventricular function (EF 35%-49%)[4] |
| | Changing pattern of or new development of angina pectoris |
| High | Prior myocardial infarction or infarct involving $\geq$ 35% of left ventricle[3,4,10,12,13] |
| | EF < 35% at rest[5] |
| | Fall in exercise systolic blood pressure or failure of systolic blood pressure to rise more than 10 mm Hg on exercise tolerance test[5,6,8,12] |
| | Persistent or recurrent ischemic pain 24 hours or more after hospital admission[5,12] |
| | Functional capacity < 5 METs[7,9] with hypotensive blood pressure response or $\geq$ 1 mm ST-segment depression[13] |
| | Congestive heart failure syndrome in hospital[3,4,5] |
| | $\geq$ 2 mm ST-segment depression at peak heart rate $\leq$ 135 bpm[4,5] |
| | High-grade ventricular ectopy[18] |

*Note.* 1 MET = 3.5 ml $O_2$/kg/min; EF = ejection fraction.

## Continuous ECG Monitoring During Phase II Cardiac Exercise Therapy: Rationale and Recommendations

The need for routine, continuous electrocardiographic (ECG) monitoring of *all* patients during immediate post-hospital exercise-based cardiac rehabilitation programs (Phase II) is controversial,[20,21] and it is this program component that has a major cost impact.[22,23]

According to a recent survey,[24] 87% of an expert panel of physicians stated that the use of telemetry ECG monitoring is established as essential to the safety and effectiveness of a prescribed regimen of exercise in coronary rehabilitation. However, there have been no controlled studies comparing the safety of exercise training conducted with on-

**Supervision and monitoring should be guided by the patient's level of risk.**

**The need for continuous, extended ECG monitoring of *all* patients during Phase II is controversial.**

site medical supervision, with and without continuous ECG monitoring.

Haskell[25] reported that the sudden death rate in programs that provided continuous ECG monitoring was less than one fourth the rate of programs that did not. However, it was acknowledged that other program characteristics (e.g., closer medical supervision, lower exercise intensity) could have accounted for these differing rates. On the other hand, Van Camp and Peterson[26] reported no statistically significant difference in the frequency of cardiovascular complications in programs that used continuous ECG monitoring versus those that monitored intermittently or "as needed."

Those that question the need for extended, continuous ECG monitoring during Phase II cardiac rehabilitation emphasize that it is costly,[22,23] that only selected patients benefit from it regarding adjustments in their medical management,[23,27] and that there is no relation between cardiovascular complications during exercise and the time post-event.[25,28-30] In addition, the safety and efficacy of Phase II cardiac rehabilitation has, in some patients, been demonstrated with a six-session protocol.[31]

In summary, it appears that formal cardiac rehabilitation programs should involve risk factor counseling plus a supervised exercise program, with or without continuous ECG monitoring. All cardiac exercise programs should, of course, also include the monitoring of blood pressure and heart rate palpation to insure that the participant is exercising within a safe and effective intensity range. ECG-monitored programs generally include three exercise sessions per week for up to 12 weeks. The triaging of patients into ECG-monitored or non-monitored programs can be performed using the level of risk stratification in which the patient has been placed. The following list provides the criteria for electrocardiographic monitoring advocated by the American College of Cardiology/American Heart Association Subcommittee on Cardiac Rehabilitation.[32] Additional studies examining the safety and efficacy of ECG monitoring in cardiac rehabilitation are necessary if guidelines are to be refined beyond these general recommendations.

*Characteristics of Patients Most Likely to Benefit*
*From Continuous ECG Monitoring During Cardiac Rehabilitation**

1. Severely depressed left ventricular function (ejection fraction below 30%)
2. Resting complex ventricular arrhythmia
3. Ventricular arrhythmias appearing or increasing with exercise
4. Decrease in systolic blood pressure with exercise
5. Survivors of sudden cardiac death
6. Survivors of myocardial infarction complicated by congestive heart failure, cardiogenic shock, and/or serious ventricular arrhythmias
7. Severe coronary artery disease and marked exercise-induced ischemia (ST-segment depression $\geq$ 2 mm)
8. Inability to self-monitor heart rate because of physical or intellectual impairment

---

*Note. Adapted with permission from the American College of Cardiology (*Journal of the American College of Cardiology*, Vol. 7, No. 2, February, p. 453, 1986).

**Formal cardiac rehabilitation programs should involve risk factor counseling plus a supervised exercise program.**

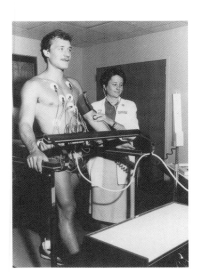

# References

1. O'Connor GT, Buring JE, Yusuf S, Goldhaber SZ, Olmstead EM, Paffenbarger RS, Hennekens, CH. An overview of randomized trials of rehabilitation with exercise after myocardial infarction. *Circulation*. 1989;80:234-244.

2. Oldridge NB, Guyatt GH, Fischer ME, Rimm AA. Cardiac rehabilitation after myocardial infarction. Combined experience of randomized clinical trials. *JAMA*. 1988;260:945-950.

3. Beller GA, Gibson RS. Risk stratification after myocardial infarction. *Mod Concepts Cardiovasc Dis*. 1986;55(2):5-10.

4. DeBusk RF, Blomqvist G, Kouchoukos NT, et al. Identification and treatment of low risk patients after acute myocardial infarction and coronary artery bypass graft surgery. *N Eng J Med*. 1986;314(3): 161-166.

5. DeBusk RF, Kraemer HC, Nash E. Stepwise risk stratification soon after acute myocardial infarction. *Am J Cardiol*. 1983;52:1161-1166.

6. Hammermeister KE, DeRouen TA, Dodge HT. Variables predictive of survival in patients with coronary disease: selection of univariate and multivariate analyses from clinical, electrocardiographic, exercise, angiographic and quantitative angiographic evaluation. *Circulation*. 1979;59(3):421-430.

7. Hung J, Goris ML, Nash E, Kraemer HC, DeBusk RF. Comparative value of maximal treadmill testing, exercise thallium myocardial perfusion scintigraphy, and exercise radionuclide ventriculography for distinguishing high and low risk patients soon after myocardial infarction. *Am J Cardiol*. 1984;53:1221-1227.

8. Krone RJ, Gillespie JA, Weld FM, Miller JP, Moss A. Low level exercise testing after myocardial infarction: usefulness in enhancing clinical risk stratification. *Circulation*. 1985;71(1):80-89.

9. McNeer JF, Margolis JR, Lee KL, et al. Role of the exercise test in evaluating patients for ischemic heart disease. *Circulation*. 1978; 57(1):64-70.

10. Madsen EB, Gilpin E, Henning H, et al. Prediction of late mortality after myocardial infarction from variables measured at different times during hospitalization. *Am J Cardiol*. 1984;53:47-54.

11. The Multicenter Post Infarction Research Group. Risk stratification and survival after myocardial infarction. *N Engl J Med*. 1983; 309(6):331-336.

12. Waters DD, Bosch X, Bouchard A, et al. Comparison of clinical variables and variables derived from a limited predischarge exercise test as predictors of early and late mortality after myocardial infarction. *J Am Coll Cardiol*. 1985;5(1):1-8.

13. Weiner DA, Ryan TJ, McCabe CH, et al. Value of exercise test in determining the risk classification in the response to coronary artery bypass grafting in three vessel coronary artery disease: a report from the CASS registry. *Am J Cardiol*. 1987;60(4):262-266.

14. Greenland P, Chu J. Position paper: cardiac rehabilitation services. *Ann Intern Med*. 1988;109:671-673.

15. Jugdutt BI, Michorowski BL, Kappagoda CT. Exercise training after anterior Q wave myocardial infarction: importance of regional left

ventricular function and topography. *J Am Coll Cardiol.* 1988;12: 362-372.

16. Ross J, Gilpin EA, Madsen EB, et al. A decision scheme for coronary angiography after acute myocardial infarction. *Circulation.* 1989;79:292-303.

17. Nicod P, Gilpin E, Dittrich H, et al. Short- and long-term clinical outcome after Q-wave and non-Q-wave myocardial infarction in a large patient population. *Circulation.* 1989;79:528-536.

18. Bigger JT, Fleiss JL, Kleiger R, et al. The relationships among ventricular arrhythmia, left ventricular dysfunction and mortality in the first two years after myocardial infarction. *Circulation.* 1984;69:250-258.

19. Huang D, Ades PA, Weaver S. Cardiac rehospitalization and costs are reduced following cardiac rehabilitation. *Circulation.* 1989;80(suppl II):II-610.

20. Greenland P, Chu JS. Efficacy of cardiac rehabilitation services with emphasis on patients after myocardial infarction. *Ann Intern Med.* 1988;109:650-663.

21. Feigenbaum E, Carter E. *Cardiac Rehabilitation Services.* Washington, DC: U.S. Department of Health and Human Services; 1987. Health Technology Assessment Report (No. 6).

22. Byl N, Reed P, Franklin B, Gordon S. Cost of phase II cardiac rehabilitation: implications regarding ECG-monitoring practices. *Circulation.* 1988;78:S2-136.

23. Greenland P, Pomilla PV. ECG monitoring in cardiac rehabilitation: is it needed? *Phys Sportsmed.* 1989;17:75-82.

24. Diagnostic and therapeutic technology assessment (DATTA): coronary rehabilitation services. *JAMA.* 1987;258:1959-1962.

25. Haskell WL. Cardiovascular complications during exercise training of cardiac patients. *Circulation.* 1978;57:920-924.

26. Van Camp SP, Peterson RA. Cardiovascular complications of outpatient cardiac rehabilitation programs. *JAMA.* 1986;256: 1160-1163.

27. Mitchell M, Franklin B, Johnson S, et al. Cardiac exercise programs: role of continuous electrocardiographic monitoring. *Arch Phys Med Rehabil.* 1984;65:463-466.

28. Mead WF, Pyfer HR, Trombold JC, et al. Successful resuscitation of two near simultaneous cases of cardiac arrest with a review of fifteen cases occurring during supervised exercise. *Circulation.* 1976;53:187-189.

29. Fletcher GF, Cantwell JD. Ventricular fibrillation in a medically supervised cardiac exercise program: clinical, angiographic, and surgical correlations. *JAMA.* 1979;238:2627-2639.

30. Hossack KF, Hartwig R. Cardiac arrest associated with supervised cardiac rehabilitation. *J Cardiac Rehab.* 1982;2:402-408.

31. Fletcher BJ, Thiel J, Fletcher GF. Phase II intensive monitored cardiac rehabilitation for coronary artery disease and coronary risk factors—a six-session protocol. *Am J Cardiol.* 1986;57:751-756.

32. American College of Cardiology Position Report on Cardiac Rehabilitation. *J Am Coll Cardiol.* 1986;7:451-453.

*Chapter 2*

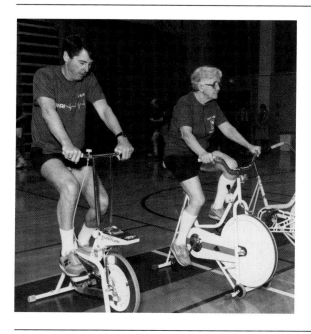

# *Graded Exercise Testing and Exercise Prescription*

This chapter includes selected references and procedures for graded exercise testing and exercise prescription. Graded exercise testing is the recommended precursor to formulating the exercise prescription. The initial exercise prescription (e.g., after acute myocardial infarction) serves to progress the patient toward resuming activities of daily living. Continued exercise training can further augment physical work capacity, increasing functional reserves.

## Graded Exercise Testing

The recommended procedures for administering graded exercise tests (GXTs) are those outlined by the American College of Sports Medicine (ACSM) guidelines.[1] Additional information relative to standards of practice in exercise testing may be obtained from the American Heart Association (AHA).[2,3] A more thorough review of clinical perspectives and physiological principles forming the basis of GXTs may be found

> The exercise prescription should be based on the physiologic responses to graded exercise testing.

in several different references;[4-9] however, this list need not be considered all-inclusive.

## Contraindications to Exercise Testing

There are certain patients for whom the risks of exercise testing may outweigh the potential information that might be gained. These individuals should simply not be tested. There are other individuals whose medical conditions increase the risk of treadmill or cycle ergometer testing. It is important in these circumstances for the referring physician and test administrator to carefully consider the anticipated benefits and determine that these outweigh the risks.

The absolute and relative contraindications for maximal exercise testing are described elsewhere.[1] Some of these contraindications may not apply in circumstances where an individual is being tested for specific reasons after a myocardial infarction, coronary revascularization surgery, or percutaneous transluminal coronary angioplasty. For example, exercise testing of the convalescing patient with "uncomplicated" myocardial infarction is now often used not only to assess a patient's functional status, but as a diagnostic, prognostic, and therapeutic guide. Whether the predischarge exercise test should be symptom-limited, or stopped when an arbitrary "submaximal" endpoint is achieved, is still controversial.

## Exercise Training and Prescription

The most effective exercises for aerobic exercise training employ large muscle groups, are maintained continuously, and are rhythmical and aerobic in nature; examples include: walking, jogging (in place or moving), running, stationary or outdoor bicycling, swimming, skipping rope, rowing, climbing stairs, and stepping on and off a bench. Because of the relative consistency of energy expenditure in walking, jogging, and cycling, these activities lend themselves particularly well to exercise prescription, offering comparable cardiorespiratory improvements when the exercise frequency, intensity, and duration are equated. Other activities commonly used in conditioning programs for cardiac patients include calisthenics, particularly those involving sustained total body movement; arm exercise; and weight training. The latter is a particularly important option, since traditional aerobic conditioning regimens often fail to accommodate participants who have an interest in improving muscular strength and endurance.

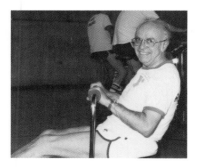

Although cardiac exercise programs have traditionally emphasized lower extremity dynamic aerobic exercise, recent research studies suggest that complementary weight training programs are safe for selected patients with coronary artery disease. Weight training guidelines for healthy adults and low-risk cardiac patients are shown in the following list, with specific reference to the appropriate number of sets and repetitions, progression, proper breathing technique, and safety concerns.

20. Haskell WL. Safety of outpatient cardiac exercise programs: issues regarding medical supervision. In: Franklin BA, Rubenfire M, eds. *Symposium on Cardiac Rehabilitation (Clinics in Sports Medicine)*. Philadelphia: WB Saunders; 1984:455-469.

21. Ehsani AA, Heath GW, Hagberg JM, et al. Effects of 12 months of intense exercise training on ischemic ST-segment depression in patients with coronary artery disease. *Circulation*. 1981;64: 1116-1124.

22. Hagberg JM, Ehsani AA, Holloszy JO. Effect of 12 months of intensive exercise training on stroke volume in patients with coronary artery disease. *Circulation*. 1983;67:1194-1199.

23. Hossack KF, Hartwig R. Cardiac arrest associated with supervised cardiac rehabilitation. *J Cardiac Rehab*. 1982;2:402-408.

# Chapter 3

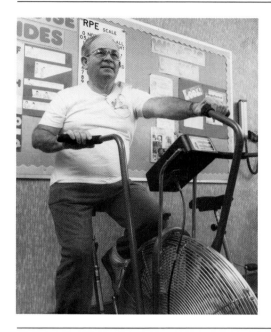

# *Patient Assessment and Educational Programming*

This chapter reflects an assessment of the cardiac patient's needs for lifestyle and behavioral change. It considers the assessment as well as the expected outcomes which are in accordance with the recommendations of the Joint Commission on Accreditation of Healthcare Organizations (JCAHO). Additionally, guidelines for educational programming for all levels/phases of cardiac rehabilitation are included.

## Inpatient, Immediate Post-Hospital, Extended Outpatient, and Maintenance Cardiac Rehabilitation Programming

Patients enter cardiac rehabilitation programs by physician referral according to the previously described stages and stratification models. After initial assessment, a patient clinical profile is established, appropriate programs designed to address specific pathological, psychological, social, and physical characteristics are outlined, and expected outcomes from the program are defined.

**Initiating behavior change through education of the patient is one of the primary goals of cardiac rehabilitation.**

Initiating behavior change through education of the patient is one of the primary goals of cardiac rehabilitation. The educational program should involve the physician, nurse, exercise specialist, nutritionist, psychologist, and other members of the health care team. The objective is the integration of lifestyle behaviors such as diet, exercise, smoking cessation, and stress management to effect positive physical and psychosocial well-being. A model for eliciting health promoting behaviors through education may be structured after the theoretical rationale of Bandura and others,[1-3] which postulates that desired behavioral outcomes will result from a selected behavioral construct, and that these desired outcomes occur when the client believes that he or she is able to learn and perform the desired behavior.

**Programs of behavior change and risk-factor modification should be based on "outcome" theory.**

A program of behavior change and risk-factor modification that is based on "outcome" theory will help the client

- identify the problem and turn it into a positive outcome;
- break down the outcome into manageable target outcomes;
- establish belief that the outcomes, when achieved, will produce the desired results;
- identify resources to learn the necessary skills; and
- develop an appropriate plan of action.[1]

Application of outcome-expectation models should occur at each phase of cardiac rehabilitation, with a new assessment of the characteristic (where the patient is at this moment) and establishment of new goals appropriate to where the patient should be in the continuum of her or his recovery.

The assessment is a delineation of conditions, behaviors, physical characteristics, and so forth, of the patient, with the baseline indicated by where he or she is right now. Levels of outcome are determined using a three-level model as follows:

Level 1 (A): Best anticipated success—the ideal.

Level 2 (B): Expected level of treatment success—the real.

Level 3 (C): The most unfavorable outcome possible—no change, increased abuse.[4-6]

**Goals have no specific, verifiable outcomes or deadlines. Objectives are measurable across time.**

Goals are broad statements of intention with no definable, specific, verifiable outcomes or deadlines. Objectives are statements of intent that specify results and outcomes according to time lines. Objectives are measurable.

In establishing the outcome objectives, there are no clear-cut guidelines from the literature relative to whatever is the most desirable endpoint—for instance, counting the number of cigarettes smoked or not smoked, or pounds lost or not lost; or establishing a scale of behavioral adaptation/acceptance (e.g., has no understanding/is working on it/has a complete understanding). It is recommended that the patient be the one who sets the objective, in conjunction with the physician and cardiac rehabilitation staff, and also determines what is the measurable proof that the outcome has been achieved.[1]

A specific programming design is illustrated in Table 3.1. However, it need not be limited to these examples.

**Table 3.1 Design for Patient Assessment, Recommended Program, and Expected Outcome Measures**

| Patient assessment and profile | Program | Expected outcome |
|---|---|---|
| Recent open chest or heart surgery (CABG, valve, AICD, pacemaker, etc.) as determined by patient medical records | Patient education program including information on the disease process, treatment and risk-factor education, activity guidelines, sexual activity, medications, and return to work | Self-care; increased understanding of surgically related concerns and improved quality of life |
| Recent diagnosis of CAD/MI or its treatment or sequelae, e.g., cath, PTCA, arrhythmia, CHF, as determined by patient medical records | Patient education program including information on the disease process, signs and symptoms, treatment options, risk factors, activity guidelines, sexual activity, medications, and return to work | Self-care; increased understanding of coronary artery disease (CAD)–related concerns and improved quality of life |
| Reduced activity level, decreased functional capacity, or sedentary lifestyle as determined by a medical history or a graded exercise test, with or without oxygen-consumption measurements | Individualized exercise program based on risk stratification: <br> • monitored <br> • unmonitored, supervised <br> • home exercise program and education | Increase in activity level and functional capacity, attainment of an improved level of fitness and/or regular exercise participation |
| Tobacco use or abuse as determined by patient or family report, CO monitoring, or isothiocyanide saliva testing | Smoking cessation program | Reduction or cessation of smoking |
| Any abnormality in blood lipids and/or lipoproteins as manifested by increased total cholesterol or LDL-C, and/or triglycerides, and/or reduced HDL-cholesterol as determined by fasting draw (for LDL-C, TG, HDL-C) and confirmed by repeat measurement | Dietary lipid/modification and medical intervention program in accordance with National Cholesterol Education Program (NCEP) guidelines: weight reduction program and/or exercise program when appropriate | Alteration toward or attainment of appropriate blood lipid and lipoprotein levels as set forth in the NCEP guidelines |
| Hypertension as determined by blood pressure sphygmomanometry | Hypertension management program including medical intervention and education in accordance with the National High Blood Pressure Education Program (NHBPEP) guidelines: weight reduction, stress management, dietary modification, and/or exercise programs when appropriate | Decreased blood pressure or attainment of appropriate blood pressure as set forth in the NHBPEP guidelines, and reduction or elimination of blood pressure medication |
| Excess body weight or relative fatness as determined by scale, body mass index, skinfold calipers, or hydrostatic weighing | Dietary weight reduction program and/or exercise program in accordance with the American Dietetic Association (ADA) guidelines | Reduction in body weight and fat stores and attainment of desirable body weight |
| High stress levels and/or inappropriate response to stress as determined by patient or family report, stress assessment tools, or psychological evaluation | Stress management program | Reduction in stress and/or inappropriate response to stress |

*(Cont.)*

**Table 3.1  (Continued)**

| Patient assessment and profile | Program | Expected outcome |
| --- | --- | --- |
| Recent onset of elevated or poorly controlled blood glucose levels as determined by fasting blood draw | Diabetes education and medical intervention program in accordance with the American Diabetes Association (ADA) guidelines; dietary modification, exercise, and/or weight reduction programs when appropriate | Controlled blood glucose levels |
| Limitation in work status due to cardiovascular medical conditions | Work hardening program and vocational rehabilitation counseling with a return to work assessment; stress management and/or exercise program when appropriate | Return to work if appropriate |
| Alcohol abuse as determined by patient or family report or by psychological evaluation | Alcohol abuse program including spouse and family therapy | Appropriate alcohol use or abstinence and appropriate family interaction |
| Psychological disorders (anxiety, depression, phobias, aggressive behavior, etc.) as determined by patient or family report or by psychological/psychiatric evaluation | Individualized and/or group therapy | Improved psychological profile and functioning |
| Neuropsychological disorders (memory loss, confusion, etc.) as determined by patient or family report or by neuropsychological evaluation | Neurological or neuropsychological referral and intervention and therapy | Improved neuropsychological profile and functioning |

**Those who provide educational counseling services need to know principles of behavior, behavior change, and adult learning.**

## Educational Services

Application of the following recommendations with regard to education of the cardiac patient begins with an understanding of the principles of behavior, behavior change, and adult learning. The cardiac rehabilitation staff involved in patient education and risk-factor reduction should have a thorough understanding of the following principles:

I.  Teaching strategies utilizing methods based on the principles of adult education, behavior change, and learning.
    A.  Antecedents and readiness[1,2,7,8]
        1.  Information and knowledge
        2.  Instructions and values
        3.  Role models and beliefs
        4.  Previous experience and skills
        5.  Incentives and disincentives
        6.  Locus of control—extrinsic and intrinsic motivation
    B.  Adoption[1,2,8,9]
        1.  Self-efficacy
        2.  Behavioral intention
        3.  Behavior

C. Maintenance[5,9-13]
    1. Lapse and relapse prevention
    2. Reinforcement
    3. Monitoring and self-report strategies
    4. Contracting

Knowledge is the gathering of cognitive information in order to understand an event, process, or phenomenon. When one has knowledge or understanding, one is able to perceive the relationships among the facts relative to the event, process, or phenomenon. Knowledge, education, and experience are the essentials of behavior change. Education is a critical part of the motivation to behavior change and "living well," as alterations in beliefs and attitudes are made based on what is known.[1]

II. It is recommended that educational services be developed using the following principles and resources.
    A. Categorize and apply educational information based upon patient needs and available resources:
        1. What the patient can learn and do on her or his own
        2. What is available for self-learning/teaching
            a. Pamphlets
            b. Books
            c. Audio cassettes
            d. Video cassettes
            e. Developed interactive training programs
        3. Education and intervention that only developed programs can provide

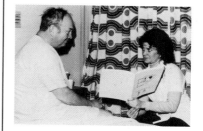

Information varies relative to the reading and comprehension level of the patient. Current national statistics indicate that 13% of high school seniors do not read above a sixth-grade level and that one in seven American adults does not read above a fourth-grade level.[14,15] All written materials should be evaluated for clarity and appropriate reading level for the user population. Utilizing a readability formula is one way of ensuring this.[16-20]

    B. Develop programs that follow established national standards and guidelines where available.
        1. National Institute of Health
        2. National Cholesterol Education Program
        3. National High Blood Pressure Education Program
        4. American Diabetes Association
        5. American Lung Association
        6. American College of Sports Medicine Position Statements
        7. American Heart Association
        8. American Cancer Society
        9. National Weight Control Resource Directory
        10. Sports and Cardiovascular Nutritionists of the American Dietetic Association
        11. Others as deemed appropriate

Cardiac rehabilitation programs should follow established national guidelines when possible.

**Programs may include discussion of risk factors, medications, signs and symptoms, work-related concerns, psychosocial problems, physiology, and safety.**

C. Develop program guidelines that include expected outcomes as part of the objectives.
   1. Evaluation of performance by patient (see pages 28 to 31)
   2. Evaluation of service[21-25]

When developing content areas for the instructive materials to be used in patient and family education, it is essential to use what has been (a) developed by national guidelines and programs, (b) developed and approved by the physicians and education departments of your state and local societies, and finally (c) approved by your hospital's medical committee and board of trustees. In all cases, local, regional, and national consensus in information will increase adherence to recommended behaviors for enhanced health and quality of life.

Components of educational, vocational, and psychological programs should include but not be limited to the following:

III. Program content.
   A. Risk factors
      1. Blood pressure management: established program according to the National High Blood Pressure Education Program (NHBPEP) guidelines[26]
      2. Lipid management: established program according to the National Cholesterol Education Program guidelines[27]
      3. Smoking cessation: according to standards of behavior change for addictive behaviors[1,2,5,7-13,28]
      4. Management of diabetes: according to guidelines established by the American Dietetic Association and American Diabetes Association
      5. Weight control: Sports and Cardiovascular Nutritionists (SCAN), American Dietetic Association (ADA), Society for Nutrition Education (SNE), and Office of Disease Prevention and Health Promotion resource directories[29-33]
      6. Stress management: utilization of biofeedback, professional programs, and classes, through referral or seminar
      7. Sedentary lifestyle: education resources based on research studies of physical activity in health and disease states[34-42] (refer to the section on exercise prescription for programming)
   B. Medication education
      1. Adherence
      2. Compliance
      3. Interaction—Food, Drug, Exercise, Sexuality
      4. Side effects
   C. Signs and symptoms
      1. Myocardial infarction and angina
      2. Congestive heart failure
      3. Hypo- and hyperglycemia
      4. Other cardiovascular patients
         a. Transplant
         b. Valve replacement

**Patients should be taught about the interaction of foods, drugs, exercise, and sexuality.**

c. Pacemaker/AICD
d. Cardiomyopathy
5. Multiple disease interaction
D. Vocational programs
1. Referral system to state vocational rehabilitation counselors
2. Program of return-to-work assessment
3. Identification of resources for assistance in the community
E. Psychosocial intervention
1. It is recognized that psychological dysfunction may be a problem for the patient with heart disease. A referral system should be made available for those patients and families having difficulty in coping with the disease, lifestyle changes, loss, depression, and related feelings.
2. Sexual function should be assessed, and the gradual, safe return to normal sexual activity should be stressed. Referral for sexual problems should be made to the appropriate educational or counseling agency.
F. Anatomy and physiology, exercise physiology, pathophysiology[43]
1. Programs of education to help the patient and family understand
a. The atherosclerotic process[44]
b. Normal versus pathological anatomy
c. Normal and abnormal exercise responses
d. Exercise prescription
1. Frequency, intensity, duration, mode
2. Perceived exertion
e. Home exercise[45]
f. Overuse symptoms and signs of injury
G. Safety
1. CPR training: American Heart Association
2. Environmental understanding
a. Heat and cold
b. Humidity
c. Wind chill
d. Altitude

**The early return to work of cardiac patients based on an occupational evaluation is associated with important socio-economic benefits.**

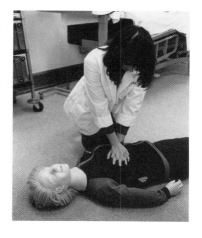

# References

1. Girdano DA, Dusek DE. *Changing Health Behavior*. Scottsdale, AZ: Gorsuch Scarisbrick; 1988.
2. Bandura A. Self-efficacy: toward a unifying theory of behavioral change. *Psychol Rev.* 1977;84:191-215.
3. Bandura A. *Social Learning Theory*. Englewood Cliffs, NJ: Prentice-Hall; 1977.
4. LaFerriere L, Calsyn R. Goal attainment scaling as an adjunct to counseling. *Journal of Counseling Psychology.* 1976;23:22-27.
5. Kiresuk TJ, Sherman RE. Goal attainment scaling: a general

method for evaluating comprehensive community mental health programs. *Community Ment Health J.* 1968;4:443-453.

6. Kiresuk TJ. Basic goal attainment scaling procedures. *P.E.P. Report 1969-1973.* Minneapolis: Program Evaluation Resource Center; 1974: chapter 1.

7. Taylor CB, Miller NH, Flora J. Principles of Behavior Change. In: Blair SN, Painter P, Pate RR, Smith LK, Taylor RB, eds. *Resource Manual for Guidelines For Exercise Testing and Prescription.* Philadelphia: Lea & Febiger; 1988.

8. Insel PM, Roth WT. *Core Concepts in Health.* Palo Alto, CA: Mayfield; 1985.

9. Marlatt GA, Gordon JR. *Relapse Prevention: Maintenance Strategies in the Treatment of Addictive Behaviors.* New York: Guilford Press; 1985.

10. Donovan DM, Marlatt GA. *Assessment of Addictive Behaviors.* New York: Guilford Press; 1988.

11. Brownell KD, Marlatt GA, Lictenstein E, Wilson TG. Understanding and preventing relapse. *Am Psychol.* 1986;41:765-782.

12. Schacter S. Recidivism and self-cure of smoking and obesity. *Am Psychol.* 1982;37:436-444.

13. Childers JH, Guyton R. Health counseling: an interdisciplinary approach. *Health Educ.* 1985;16(3):7-9.

14. National Collaboration for Youth. Growing up isn't easy for many. *USA Today.* September 14, 1989;11A.

15. Stoffer H. Ranks of illiterates are continuing to swell. *Pittsburgh Post-Gazette.* September 8, 1989;1.

16. U.S. Department of Health and Human Services. *Pretesting in Health Communications: Methods, Examples, and Resources for Improving Health Messages and Materials.* Bethesda, MD: NIH, NCI; Dec. 1982. NIH Publication No. 83-1493.

17. Dale E, Chale JS. A formula for predicting readability. *Educ Res Bull.* 1948;27:11-20.

18. Fry E. A readability formula that saves time. *J Reading.* 1968;11: 513-516.

19. Flesch R. A new readability yardstick. *J Appl Psychol.* 1948;32: 221-233.

20. McLaughlin G. SMOC grading—a new readability formula. *J Reading.* 1969;5:639-646.

21. Blodgett C, Perkarik G. Program evaluation in cardiac rehabilitation I: overview of evaluation issues. *J Cardiopul Rehab.* 1987; 7(7):316-323.

22. Posavic EJ, Carey RG. *Program Evaluation: Methods and Case Studies.* Englewood Cliffs, NJ: Prentice-Hall; 1985.

23. Windsor RA, Baranowski T, Clark N, Cutter G. *Evaluation of Health Promotion and Education Programs.* Palo Alto, CA: Mayfield Publishing; 1984.

24. Blodgett C, Perkarik G. Program evaluation in cardiac rehabilitation II: outcome evaluation procedures. *J Cardiopul Rehab.* 1987;7(8):374-382.

25. Blodgett C, Perkarik G. Program evaluation in cardiac rehabilitation III: utilization assessment. *J Cardiopul Rehab.* 1987;7(9):410-414.

26. 1988 Joint National Committee. The 1988 Report of the Joint Na-

tional Committee on Detection, Evaluation and Treatment of High Blood Pressure. *Arch Intern Med.* 1988;148:1023-1038.

27. The Expert Panel. Report of the National Cholesterol Education Expert Panel on Detection, Evaluation, and Treatment of High Blood Cholesterol in Adults. *Arch Intern Med.* 1988;148:36-69.

28. Pinto RP, Morrell EM. Current approaches and future trends in smoking cessation programs. *J Mental Health Counseling.* 1988; 10(2):95-110.

29. Rock CL, Coulston AM. Weight-control approaches: a review by the California Dietetic Association. *J Am Diet Assoc.* 1988;88:44.

30. Weinsier RL, Wadden TA, Ritenbaugh C, et al. Recommended therapeutic guidelines for professional weight control programs. *Am J Clin Nutr.* 1984;40: 865-872.

31. Berkowitz SA, ed. *National Weight Control Resource Directory.* Oakland, CA: Society for Nutrition Education; 1988.

32. Council on Scientific Affairs. Treatment of obesity in adults. *JAMA.* 1988;260:2547-2551.

33. Kris-Etherton PM, ed. *The SCAN Cardiovascular Practice Manual.* Chicago: American Dietetic Association; 1989.

34. Powell KE, Thompson PD, Caspersen CJ, Kendrick JS. Physical activity and the incidence of coronary heart disease. *Annu Rev Public Health.* 1987;8:253-287.

35. Editorial: Progress in chronic disease prevention. Protective effect of physical activity on coronary heart disease. *MMWR.* 1987; 36:426-430.

36. Sebrechts CP, Klein JL, Ahnve S, Froelicher VF, Ashburn WL. Myocardial perfusion changes following 1 year of exercise training assessed by thallium-201 circumferential count profiles. *Am Heart J.* 1986;112:1217-1225.

37. Leon AS, Connett J, Jacobs DR, Rauramaa R. Leisure-time physical activity levels and risk of coronary heart disease and death. *JAMA.* 1987;258:2388-2395.

38. Ekelund LG, Haskell WL, Johnson JL, et al. Physical fitness as a predictor of cardiovascular mortality in asymptomatic North American men. *N Engl J Med.* 1988;319:1379-1384.

39. Slattery ML, Jacobs DR, Nichaman MZ. Leisure time physical activity and coronary heart disease death. The U.S. Railroad Study. *Circulation.* 1989;79:304-311.

40. Evridiki IH, Koplan JP, Weinstein MC, Caspersen CJ, Warner KE. A cost-effectiveness analysis of exercise as a health promotion activity. *Am J Public Health.* 1988;78(11):1417-1421.

41. Keeler EB, Manning WG, Newhouse JP, Sloss EM, Wasserman J. The external costs of a sedentary life-style. *Am J Public Health.* 1989;79(8):975-980.

42. Harris SS. Caspersen CJ, DeFriese GH, Estes H. Physical activity counseling for healthy adults as a primary preventive intervention in the clinical setting. *JAMA.* 1989;261(24):3590-3598.

43. Pollock M. Benefits of exercise: effect on mortality and physiological function. In: Kappagoda CT, Greenwood PV, eds. *Long-Term Management of Patients After Myocardial Infarction.* Boston: Martinus Nijhoff Publishing; 1988:189-205.

44. Raichlen JS, Healy B, Achuff SC, Pearson TA. Importance of risk

factors in the angiographic progression of coronary artery disease. *Am J Cardiol.* 1986;57:66-70.

45. Blair SN, Kohl HW, Paffenbarger RS, Clark DG, Cooper KH, Gibbons LW. Physical fitness and all-cause mortality. *JAMA.* 1989;262:2395-2401.

# Chapter 4

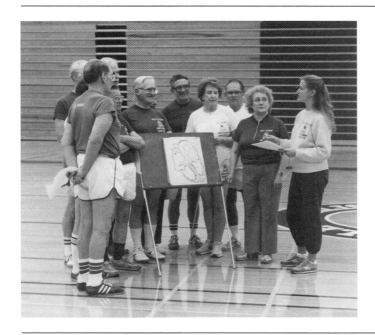

# Program Evaluation and Efficacy Measures

Recommendations in this chapter pertain to the evaluation and assessment of program components and their outcomes, as applied to the patient. Such measures can be used to assess the effectiveness of the intervention and to make changes when it appears that the program is failing to accomplish the desired outcomes.

## Assessing Program Effectiveness

Evaluation of the program should be a direct application of the existing management principles upon which the department and hospital are founded. The JCAHO provides guidelines for evaluation of services relative to their quality and appropriateness through utilization of the following:

- Collection of data relative to important aspects of care
- Assessment of information to identify problems
- Action taken on identified problems
- Evaluation of outcomes

> **Efficacy measures can be used to assess an intervention's effectiveness and to make changes when necessary.**

**There should be a complementary relationship between efficacy measures and expected outcomes.**

- Report of conclusions
- Annual reappraisal of programs to determine effectiveness[1-6]

Additionally, efficacy measures should be made on each component of the cardiac rehabilitation program to evaluate application effectiveness. A relationship of these measures with expected outcomes of individualized patient programming should exist. Table 4.1 lists recommended efficacy measures, but these need not be considered all-inclusive.

**Table 4.1   Suggested Efficacy Measures for Program Evaluation**

| Program | Efficacy Measures |
| --- | --- |
| Patient education program for recent heart surgery and for recent diagnosis of CAD/MI or its nonsurgical treatment | Percentage of participants completing program? Percentage of sessions attended? Percentage improvement in pre- versus posttest knowledge? Percentage answers correct on posttest? |
| | Percentage of participants returning to self-care activities at similar or improved level of performance within 1 month? 3 months? 6 months post hospital discharge? |
| | Percentage of participants returning to sexual activity at similar or improved level of performance within 1 month? 3 months? 6 months post hospital discharge? |
| | Average participant score on level of understanding pre and post program? Average difference? |
| | Average participant score on level of adaptation at similar or improved level of performance within 1 month? 3 months? 6 months post hospital discharge? |
| Individualized exercise program | In-hospital: Percentage of patients participating in minimum of one? three? five total exercise sessions? |
| | Percentage of patients who demonstrated functional improvements (progressed ambulation) during participation in the exercise program? |
| | Percentage of exercise sessions in which exertion-related complications required medical attention for the patient? |
| | Average number of sessions attended per patient? Average number of education sessions attended per patient? |
| | Post-hospital maintenance: Percentage of participants completing program? Percentage of the total sessions attended? |
| | Percentage of participants exercising a minimum of three times per week (at home or in a structured program)? |
| | Percentage of patients increasing functional capacity after 3 months and at 1 year? Average change? |
| | Percentage of participants achieving a high, medium, or low fitness level based on national standards for age and gender? |

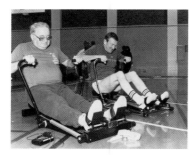

| Program | Efficacy Measures |
|---|---|
| | Percentage of patients who experienced orthopedic and/or musculoskeletal complications? |
| | Percentage of participants who withdrew from the program because of the new onset of symptoms of congestive heart failure or the worsening of baseline status in patients with congestive heart failure? |
| | Percentage of participants who experienced cardiac arrest? New or worse angina? New or worse ECG changes? Inappropriate hemodynamic responses? |
| | Percentage of participants who withdrew from program due to cardiac arrest? New or worse angina? New or worse ECG changes? Inappropriate hemodynamic responses? |
| | Percentage of patients who withdrew from program because of the new onset of symptoms of congestive heart failure or worsening baseline status in CHF patients? |
| | Percentage of participants who were successfully treated and completed program following cardiac arrest? New or worse angina? New or worse ECG changes? Inappropriate hemodynamic responses? |
| | Average level of behavior acceptance pre and post program? Average difference? |
| | Average level of behavior compliance pre and post program? Average difference? |
| Smoking cessation program | Percentage of participants completing program? Percentage of participants who dropped out at 3 months, 6 months, 1 year? Percentage of participants who reduced their smoking at 3 months, 6 months, 1 year? Average reduction? |
| | Average level of behavior acceptance preprogram to 3 months? 6 months? 1 year? Average difference? |
| | Average level of behavior compliance preprogram to 3 months? 6 months? 1 year? Average difference? |
| Lipid modification program | Percentage of participants who completed the program? Percentage of participants utilizing lipid-lowering medications? Frequency of adverse side effects? Percentage of participants with and without medications who reduced their lipid levels at 3 months? 6 months? 1 year? |
| | Percentage of participants following NCEP Step-One diet? Percentage of participants following NCEP Step-Two diet? |
| | Average entry total cholesterol, LDL, HDL, and triglycerides? Average exit total cholesterol, LDL, HDL, and triglycerides? |
| | Average change per participant at 3 months? 6 months? 1 year? Percentage of participants who achieved NCEP goals at 3 months? 6 months? 1 year? |

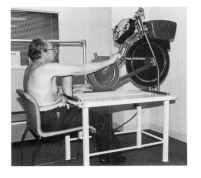

**Recording patient outcomes over time can help to measure a program's long-term success.**

**(Cont.)**

**Table 4.1  (Continued)**

| Program | Efficacy Measures |
|---------|-------------------|
| | Frequency of patients experiencing adverse or limiting side effects from lipid-lowering medications? |
| | Average level of behavior acceptance preprogram to 3 months? 6 months? 1 year? Average difference? |
| | Average level of behavior compliance preprogram to 3 months? 6 months? 1 year? Average difference? |
| Hypertension management program | Percentage of participants completing the program? Percentage of participants who reduced medication at 3 months? 6 months? 1 year? Percentage of participants who eliminated their medication at 3 months? 6 months? 1 year? Percentage of participants who achieved NHBPEP recommendations at 3 months? 6 months? 1 year? |
| | Frequency of patients experiencing adverse or limiting side effects from antihypertension medications? |
| | Average level of behavior acceptance preprogram to 3 months? 6 months? 1 year? Average difference? |
| Weight reduction program | Percentage of participants who completed the program? Percentage of patients maintaining initial weight loss at 3 months? 6 months? 1 year? |
| | Percentage of participants who achieved their weight goal within 3 months? 6 months? 1 year? |
| | Percentage of patients who have body weights $\geq$ 30% of desirable body weight? |
| | Average level of behavior acceptance preprogram to 3 months? 6 months? 1 year? Average difference? |
| | Average level of behavior compliance preprogram to 3 months? 6 months? 1 year? Average difference? |
| Stress management program | Percentage of participants completing the program? Percentage of participants reporting a significant reduction of stress at 3 months? 6 months? 1 year? |
| | Average level of behavior acceptance preprogram to 3 months? 6 months? 1 year? Average difference? |
| | Average level of behavior compliance preprogram to 3 months? 6 months? 1 year? Average difference? |
| Diabetic program | Percentage of participants completing the program? Percentage of participants maintaining glucose control within ADA guidelines at 1 month? 3 months? 1 year? |
| | Percentage of participants maintaining fasting blood glucose (FBG) within ADA guidelines at 1 month? 3 months? 1 year? |
| | Percentage of participants reducing medication dosage after 3 months? 6 months? 1 year? |
| | Average level of behavior acceptance preprogram to 3 months? 6 months? 1 year? Average difference? |
| | Average level of behavior compliance preprogram to 3 months? 6 months? 1 year? Average difference? |

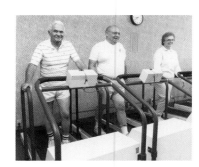

**Diabetics should follow American Diabetes Association guidelines in gaining and maintaining glucose control.**

| Program | Efficacy Measures |
| --- | --- |
| Return-to-work program | Percentage of participants on medical leave from employment who returned to work within 3 months? 6 months? 1 year after discharge? |
| | Percentage of participants referred to a state vocational rehabilitation counselor for work-related problems? |
| | Average level of behavior acceptance preprogram to 3 months? 6 months? 1 year? Average difference? |
| | Average level of behavior compliance preprogram to 3 months? 6 months? 1 year? Average difference? |
| Alcohol abuse program | Percentage of participants who completed the program? Percentage of patients whose families participated in the program? |
| | Percentage of patients who appropriately used alcohol or ceased usage after 3 months? 6 months? 1 year? |
| | Average level of behavior acceptance preprogram to 3 months? 6 months? 1 year? Average difference? |
| | Average level of behavior compliance preprogram to 3 months? 6 months? 1 year? Average difference? |
| Psychological and neuropsychological disorders therapy | Percentage of participants who improved their psychological or neuropsychological functioning at 3 months? 6 months? 1 year after discharge? |

# References

1. Blodgett C, Perkarik G. Program evaluation in cardiac rehabilitation I: overview of evaluation issues. *J Cardiopul Rehab*. 1987; 7(7):316-323.
2. Posavic EJ, Carey RG. *Program Evaluation: Methods and Case Studies*. Englewood Cliffs, NJ: Prentice-Hall; 1985.
3. Windsor RA, Baranowski T, Clark N, Cutter G. *Evaluation of Health Promotion and Education Programs*. Palo Alto, CA: Mayfield Publishing; 1984.
4. Blodgett C, Perkarik G. Program evaluation in cardiac rehabilitation II: outcome evaluation procedures. *J Cardiopul Rehab*. 1987; 7(8):374-382.
5. Blodgett C, Perkarik G. Program evaluation in cardiac rehabilitation III: utilization assessment. *J Cardiopul Rehab*. 1987;7(10): 410-414.
6. Joint Commission on Accreditation of Healthcare Organizations. *Accreditation Manual for Hospitals*. Chicago: JCAHO; 1988.

## Chapter 5

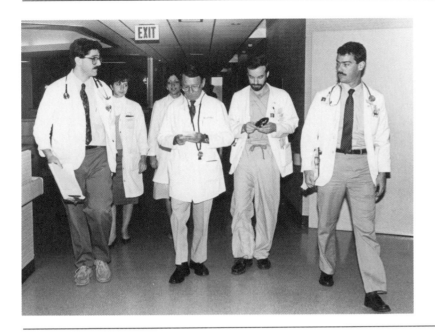

# *Personnel for Cardiovascular Rehabilitation Services*

Qualified allied health-care personnel, acting upon the referring physician's individual treatment plan, provide the services and strategies for successful rehabilitation of the cardiac patient. The collective knowledge, skills, and clinical experiences of the professional staff must reflect the multidisciplinary competencies necessary to effect the desired treatment outcomes. Depending upon individual patient needs, personnel must possess the competencies needed to guide interventions aimed at restoring functional capacity and effect favorable modification of coronary heart disease risk factors. The patient's psychological adjustment and acquisition of skills for health self-maintenance and work adjustment are also important objectives of the rehabilitation process. Staff utilization must assure safe and appropriate monitoring, instruction, and progress review for each intervention applied in the individualized plan of patient care. The clinical skills and medicolegal authority required to act in areas of care deemed critical to patient safety must be assured. Administratively, staff utilization must also be responsive to cost-containment considerations.

> The collective skills of the staff must reflect the multidisciplinary nature of cardiac rehabilitation.

In this regard, personnel should be assigned to support interventions that have been demonstrably effective and that represent definitive rehabilitative needs of the patient. Furthermore, this personnel support should be continued as long as progress toward the individualized therapeutic goals of the primary-care physician is evident.

## Competency Standards

The knowledge and technical skills required to achieve the optimal standard of care derive from several disciplines and health care professions. Primary duties include implementation and supervision of one or more physician-prescribed interventions for each patient. Working as a team, rehabilitation personnel are responsible to

- select the intervention strategies most appropriate to achieving the treatment goals for each patient;
- implement rehabilitation modules to effect the priority treatment outcomes;
- monitor the patient's participation;
- evaluate progress, adjusting strategies and treatment modalities to optimize outcome; and
- provide reports and recommendations to the primary-care physician regarding patient progress and discharge.

**Staff number, background, and specialization will vary considerably from one facility to another.**

The number, disciplinary background, and professional specialization of the personnel will vary considerably from one facility to another. Nevertheless, the collective knowledge base of the person or persons assigned to provide patient service must include a comprehensive and up-to-date understanding of cardiovascular diseases, cardiovascular nursing, cardiovascular emergency procedures, nutrition, exercise physiology, health psychology, and medical and educational strategies for CAD risk-factor management.

Both licensed and nonlicensed health care professionals may be included on the cardiovascular rehabilitation team. The professions most frequently represented in the essential staff positions include specially trained nurses, exercise physiologists, nutritionists, health educators, health psychologists, vocational rehabilitation counselors, physical therapists, corrective therapists, occupational therapists, and pharmacists, as well as physicians. Particularly in the small program with only a few individuals assigned to services on a part-time basis, it is important that the staff participate in multidisciplinary continuing education activities and/or that certification of personnel be undertaken to assure maintenance of competency standards.

**To assure maintenance of competency standards, cardiac rehabilitation personnel should regularly participate in continuing education programs and professional certifications.**

The specific competency guidelines for cardiovascular rehabilitation personnel expressed herewith are largely in agreement with standards previously published by other organizations and governmental agencies. For example, standards for education have been described by several state associations of cardiac rehabilitation, including those of California, Georgia, Massachusetts, and North Carolina,[1-4] and by the United States Health Care Finance Administration.[5] Guidelines for professional education and minimal competencies expected for certification of program directors, exercise specialists, and exercise test technologists have been developed by the American College of Sports Medicine.[6]

Minimum personnel required for a program to provide cardiovascular rehabilitation services shall include a medical director/supervising physician and a program director/coordinator. If the background and training of the program director is primarily in an allied health field such as exercise physiology, a registered nurse should be included as part of the minimum personnel. Where possible, it is recommended that the services of an exercise specialist, a physical therapist, a dietitian, a mental health professional, a vocational rehabilitation counselor, a health educator, an occupational therapist, and a pharmacist also be provided.

All personnel must possess current certification in Basic Life Support (BLS) from the American Heart Association (AHA) or equivalent. At least one person, with current certification of the AHA in Advanced Cardiac Life Support (ACLS) and the medicolegal authority to provide such care, shall be present whenever directly supervised rehabilitative exercise is provided for high- and intermediate-risk patients. Chapter 7 provides further clarification of the personnel requirements and performance expectations needed to provide appropriate emergency cardiac care in the cardiac rehabilitation setting.

The following outline delineates minimum standards for "core" personnel. In each case, the preferred educational standards for core staff are also indicated, as are the preferred standards for additional, recommended personnel or provision of optimal services.

**All personnel must be certified in Basic Life Support.**

I.  Minimum personnel
    A. Medical director/supervising physician
       1. Required qualifications
          a. Cardiologist, internist, or other physicians with interest and experience in cardiac rehabilitation licensed to practice in the jurisdiction and with special competence in rehabilitative care
          b. Experienced in exercise testing, prescription, and counseling
          c. Certified in ACLS, or experienced and knowledgeable in emergency procedures
       2. Preferred qualifications
          a. Board-certified cardiologist
          b. Experienced in medical supervision of cardiovascular rehabilitation services
    B. Program director/coordinator
       1. Required qualifications
          a. Bachelor's degree in an allied health field such as exercise physiology, or licensure in jurisdiction as a registered nurse
          b. Advanced knowledge of exercise physiology, nutrition, risk-factor modification strategies, counseling techniques, and uses of educational programs and technologies as applied to cardiovascular rehabilitative services
          c. Certification, experience, and training equivalent to those specified for an exercise specialist by the American

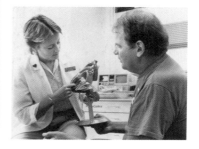

College of Sports Medicine or the advanced specialty in cardiopulmonary rehabilitation of the American Physical Therapy Association

  d. Experienced in coordination of staff and delivery of cardiovascular rehabilitation services to patients

  e. Certified in BLS or ACLS (if registered nurse)

 2. Preferred qualifications

  a. Certification, experience, and training equivalent to those specified for a program director by the American College of Sports Medicine

  b. Certified in ACLS

C. Registered Nurse

 1. Required qualifications

  a. Licensed to practice as a registered nurse in the jurisdiction

  b. Experience and/or specialty training in cardiovascular rehabilitation and critical cardiac care

  c. Basic knowledge of exercise physiology, nutrition, risk-factor modification strategies, counseling techniques, and uses of educational programs and technologies as applied to cardiovascular rehabilitative services

  d. Certified in ACLS

 2. Preferred qualifications

  a. Instructor of BLS

  b. Certification, experience, and training equivalent to those specified for an exercise specialist by the American College of Sports Medicine

II. Recommended personnel (additional)

 A. Exercise specialist

  1. Required qualifications

   a. Bachelor's degree in exercise physiology or related field

   b. Certification, experience, and training equivalent to those specified for an exercise specialist by the American College of Sports Medicine

   c. Experienced in exercise program planning, supervision, and counseling with cardiovascular rehabilitation patients

   d. Certified in BLS

  2. Preferred qualifications

   a. Master's degree in rehabilitative exercise physiology or related field

   b. Certified in ACLS

 B. Nutritionist

  1. Required qualifications

   a. Registered as a dietitian with the American Dietetic Association

   b. Experienced in practicing therapeutic dietetics in hospital and community settings, particularly in areas of lipid disorders, obesity, diabetes, and hypertension

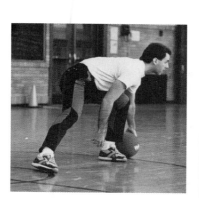

**A nutritionist should be registered as a dietitian with the American Dietetic Association.**

  c. Certified in BLS

 2. Preferred qualifications

  a. Master's degree in nutrition along with registered dietitian status with the American Dietetic Association

C. Mental health professional

 1. Required qualifications

  a. Licensed to practice in the jurisdiction as a psychological associate (monitored/supervised by licensed psychologist)

  b. Certified in BLS

 2. Preferred qualifications

  a. Licensed to practice in the jurisdiction as a psychologist or psychiatrist (physician with board certification in psychiatry)

  b. Experienced in psychological assessment, administration of health behavioral interventions, and counseling with cardiovascular rehabilitation patients

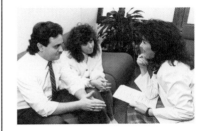

D. Health educator

 1. Required qualifications

  a. Bachelor's degree in health education or a degree as a registered nurse

  b. Experienced in providing individual and group educational programs for patient and family members to reduce coronary heart disease risk factors and promote health self-maintenance

  c. Experienced in the wide range of available technologies to provide individual health self-monitoring and promote positive health behaviors

  d. Certified in BLS

 2. Preferred qualifications

  a. Master's degree in health education

E. Vocational rehabilitation counselor

 1. Required qualifications

  a. A rehabilitation counselor, with professional education or in-service training specifically to meet cardiac rehabilitation patient needs

  b. Certified in BLS

 2. Preferred qualifications

  a. Master's degree in rehabilitation counseling

  b. Experienced in vocational counseling with cardiovascular rehabilitation patients

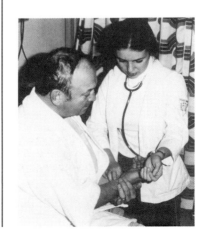

F. Physical therapist

 1. Required qualifications

  a. Licensed to practice physical therapy in the jurisdiction

  b. Experienced in the identification and physical remediation of various musculoskeletal limitations that may be present in cardiovascular rehabilitation patients

  c. Experienced in exercise program planning, supervision,

and counseling with cardiovascular rehabilitation patients*

   d. Certified in BLS

2. Preferred qualifications

   a. Certification, experience, and training equivalent to that specified for the exercise specialist of the American College of Sports Medicine or the advanced specialty in cardiopulmonary rehabilitation of the American Physical Therapy Association

   b. Certified in ACLS

G. Occupational therapist

1. Required qualifications

   a. Bachelor's degree in occupational therapy

   b. Licensed to practice in the jurisdiction, if applicable, as an occupational therapist

   c. Registered by the American Occupational Therapy Association

   d. Certified in BLS

2. Preferred qualifications

   a. Graduate degree in occupational therapy or related field

   b. Experienced in providing occupational therapy services to cardiovascular rehabilitation patients

   c. Certified in ACLS

H. Pharmacist

1. Required qualifications

   a. Graduate of an accredited school of pharmacy

   b. Licensed in the jurisdiction to practice pharmacy

   c. Certified in BLS

> Like most cardiac rehabilitation personnel, an occupational therapist should be licensed to practice in the jurisdiction.

## Utilization of Exercise Services: Considerations Regarding Safety and Supervision

The risk of serious cardiovascular complications associated with exercise is relatively low among appropriately selected rehabilitation patients.[7] Nevertheless, the likelihood of such complications is greater than among adults without coronary artery disease.[8] Patients with previous myocardial infarction who have impaired left ventricular function, significant exercise-induced ST-segment depression or angina, or threatening ventricular arrhythmias, or who have a very low or relatively high aerobic capacity, appear to be at increased risk for exercise-related cardiovascular complications. Cardiac arrest victims are also more likely to disregard appropriate warm-up and cool-down procedures or exhibit poor compliance to the prescribed training heart rate range (i.e., intensity violators). From this type of information, a profile of the high-risk patient has emerged (Table 5.1).[9-13]

The risk for cardiovascular complications and the need for a medically supervised exercise program equipped with a defibrillator and

> While the risk of exercise-related cardiovascular complications is relatively low among cardiac patients, it is significantly greater than among adults without coronary artery disease.

---

*With appropriate training and experience, the physical therapist may also serve as the exercise specialist.

**Table 5.1  Patient Characteristics Associated
With Exercise-Related Cardiovascular Complications**

| Category | Characteristic |
| --- | --- |
| Clinical status | Multiple myocardial infarctions<br>Impaired left ventricular function (ejection fraction < 30%)<br>Rest or unstable angina pectoris<br>Serious arrhythmias at rest<br>High-grade left anterior descending lesions and/or significant ($\geq$ 75% occlusion) multivessel atherosclerosis on angiography<br>Low serum potassium |
| Exercise training participation | Disregard for appropriate warm-up and cool-down<br>Consistently exceeds prescribed training heart rate |
| Exercise test data | Low or high exercise tolerance ($\leq$ 4 METs or $\geq$ 10 METs)<br>Chronotropic impairment off drugs (< 120 bpm)<br>Inotropic impairment (decrease in systolic blood pressure with increasing work loads)<br>Myocardial ischemia (angina and/or ST-segment depression $\geq$ 0.2 mV)<br>Serious cardiac arrhythmias (especially in patients with impaired left ventricular function) |
| Other | Cigarette smoker<br>Male gender |

*Note.* Adapted from References 9 through 13.

appropriate emergency drugs are held to be individual decisions made jointly by the primary-care physician and the patient. Previous reports indicate that up to 90% of all patients with exercise-related cardiac arrest are successfully resuscitated when these events occur in medically supervised and equipped programs.[7,12]

Assignment of a patient to a particular exercise regimen, requisite levels of monitoring, degree of professional supervision and the physical environment for exercise are based upon risk stratification. Clinical features characterizing the three risk categories (i.e., low, intermediate, and high) are defined elsewhere in this document. Nevertheless, *all* cardiac patients should be eligible for selected cardiac rehabilitation services (e.g., patient education, exercise therapy, risk-factor modification) to potentially prevent a deterioration in risk status over time.

Utilization of personnel to monitor and supervise exercise conditioning of high-, intermediate-, and low-risk patients is specified in Table 5.2. Exercise therapy for cardiac patients, regardless of their risk categorization, constitutes a medical procedure and, therefore, requires the availability of continuous and instantaneous ECG monitoring,[14] immediate delivery of emergency cardiac care, and substantial control by a supervising physician.

It is generally recommended that the immediate post-hospital exercise intervention program (Phase II) have a minimum staff-to-patient ratio of 1:5. Nevertheless, a second staff person should be immediately available, in case of emergency. Maintenance programs that do not involve continuous ECG monitoring should have a minimum staff-to-

**In medically supervised and equipped programs, up to 90% of all patients with exercise-related cardiac arrest are successfully resuscitated.**

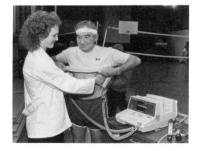

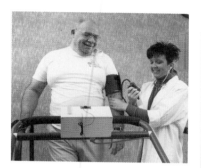

**Table 5.2  Utilization of Program Personnel in Supervision of Exercise Therapy**

| | Patient risk for exercise-related cardiovascular complications | | |
|---|---|---|---|
| Personnel category | High (hospitalized) | High/Interm. (ambulatory) | Low (maintenance) |
| Supervising physician | IA | IA/IS | IS |
| Program director/coordinator | IA | IA | IS |
| Registered nurse | IA | IA* | NA |
| Exercise specialist/leader | IA | IA | IA |

*Note.* IA = immediately available in the facility if requested by personnel authorized to visually supervise the exercising patient; IS = indirect supervision, that is, individual provides substantial influence for policy and procedure development affecting exercise services delivered to patients; also, substantially involved in planning, review of progress, and discharge assessments for each individual patient's exercise intervention; * = should be in the exercise room; NA = not applicable.

patient ratio of 1:15. Even lower staff–patient ratios and intensified monitoring techniques may be necessary if a greater proportion of the participants are intermediate-risk patients. When high-risk individuals participate in structured exercise sessions while hospitalized or as ambulatory outpatients, a supervising physician must be immediately available in the facility. Whether the intervention, determined to be a requisite of the treatment plan, involves exercise or pharmacological, nutritional, psychological, educational, or work adjustment intervention, there must be significant clinical control provided by the supervising physician. Moreover, the investment of personnel resources and the application of individualized treatment activities should be increased for the high-risk patient who requires multiple interventions.

# References

1. California Society for Cardiac Rehabilitation. *Standards for Cardiac Rehabilitation in California.* Stockton, CA: California Society for Rehabilitation; 1988.
2. American Heart Association—Georgia Affiliate. *Guidelines for Cardiac Rehabilitation Programs in Georgia.* Atlanta, GA: AHA; 1987.
3. Massachusetts Society for Cardiac Rehabilitation. *Standards for Cardiac Rehabilitation Programs.* Boston, MA: Massachusetts Society for Cardiac Rehabilitation; 1988.
4. North Carolina Cardio-Pulmonary Rehabilitation Society. *Organizational Guidelines for Cardiac Rehabilitation Programs in North Carolina.* Winston-Salem, NC: North Carolina Cardio-Pulmonary Rehabilitation Society; 1987.
5. United States Public Health Service, Health Care Finance Administration. *Comprehensive Outpatient Rehabilitation Survey Report Facility Form* (Section 488.70 Personnel Qualifications). 1982.

6. American College of Sports Medicine. *Guidelines for Exercise Testing and Prescription*. 3rd ed. Philadelphia: Lea & Febiger; 1986.

7. Van Camp SP, Peterson RA. Cardiovascular complications of outpatient cardiac rehabilitation programs. *JAMA*. 1986;256:1160-1163.

8. Cobb LA, Weaver WD. Exercise: a risk for sudden death in patients with coronary heart disease. *J Am Coll Cardiol*. 1986;7:215-219.

9. Mead WF, Pyfer HR, Trombold JC, Frederick RC. Successful resuscitation of two near simultaneous cases of cardiac arrest with a review of fifteen cases occurring during supervised exercise. *Circulation*. 1976;53:187-189.

10. Fletcher GF, Cantwell JD. Ventricular fibrillation in a medically supervised cardiac exercise program: clinical, angiographic, and surgical correlations. *JAMA*. 1977;238:2627-2629.

11. Hossack KF, Hartwig R. Cardiac arrest associated with supervised cardiac rehabilitation. *J Cardiac Rehab*. 1982;2:402-408.

12. Haskell WL. Safety of outpatient cardiac exercise programs: issues regarding medical supervision. In: Franklin BA, Rubenfire M, eds. *Symposium on Cardiac Rehabilitation (Clinics in Sports Medicine)*. Philadelphia: WB Saunders; 1984:455-469.

13. Jugdutt BI, Michorowski BL, Kappagoda CT. Exercise training after anterior Q wave myocardial infarction: importance of regional left ventricular function and topography. *J Am Coll Cardiol*. 1988;12:362-372.

14. Franklin BA, Reed PS, Gordon S, et al. Instantaneous electrocardiography: a simple screening technique for cardiac exercise programs. *Chest*. 1989;96:174-177.

# Chapter 6

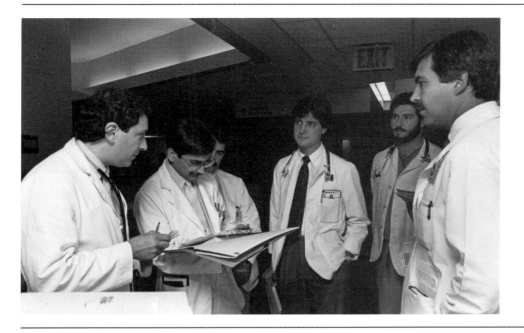

# Guidelines for Record Keeping on Participants in Cardiac Rehabilitation Programs

At each stage of cardiac rehabilitation participation, records should be kept on every participant to document both the types of interventions used and the individual's responses to them. A collection of such information is usually assembled and maintained as a patient chart. Exact specifications for forms used to collect patient data and record rehabilitation procedures vary from one institution to another. Many textbooks on cardiac rehabilitation contain suggestions and samples of how forms could be designed. Two main considerations should influence the design or selection of forms to be used with a cardiac rehabilitation program:

1. Efficiency—quick and easy use is essential to keeping records accurate and up to date.
2. Clarity—information needs to be accessible and understandable to all members of the rehabilitation team.

**Cardiac rehabilitation forms should be clear, concise, and user friendly.**

Health care professionals need to become familiar with their institution's medical record guidelines that impact the content or format of cardiac rehabilitation charts. In all cases, information contained in patient charts must be kept confidential, and patient records should be stored in a locked cabinet when not in use. Program policies should define the content, use, and storage of participant records.

## In-Hospital Rehabilitation

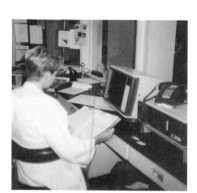

Every hospital has guidelines for the structure and use of its medical records. Often already existing forms can be used by cardiac rehabilitation team members to document the delivery to inpatients of cardiac rehabilitation (e.g., nutritional assessment sheets, physical therapy treatment sheets, nurses' notes, etc.). For ease of access and communication, some programs choose to develop specific forms to record the delivery of cardiac rehabilitation services. The most common of these are flow sheets for documenting cardiac teaching and activity progression. Such forms must be reviewed and approved by the appropriate medical records committee before they are inserted into hospital charts.

## Outpatient Rehabilitation

The content of an outpatient cardiac rehabilitation chart may vary with the type of facility in which the program is provided and with the number and type of personnel involved.

I.  Minimal documentation
    A. Past history—copies or summaries of information regarding the patient's cardiac problem and the reason the patient has been referred to the cardiac rehabilitation program
    B. Present status—forms that identify what is currently being done for the patient and how the patient is responding
    C. Future plans—written projections of rehabilitation goals and services scheduled to be provided

**Optimally, charts could include medicolegal, assessment, planning, implementation, and evaluation forms.**

II. Optimal documentation
    A. Medicolegal forms
        1. Physician's orders, including the following:
            a. Referral to program
            b. Risk-stratification placement
            c. Exercise prescription
            d. Medical orders for other procedures, treatments, referrals (e.g., lipid profiles, psychological counseling)
        2. Informed consent forms: Program participation requires an informed consent process, and a form reflecting that process must be signed by each patient. Separate consent forms are needed for each exercise stress test.
        3. Record release form: To obtain copies of a patient's records from another facility or to forward rehabilitation records

to another program, the patient must sign a release form giving her or his permission.

   B. Assessment forms

      1. A general summary of the patient's medical history, acute course, and cardiac procedures

      2. Reports of intake tests and measurements (e.g., lipid profiles, exercise stress tests)

      3. Assessment summary from each discipline involved

   C. Planning forms: A rehabilitation plan, individualized for the patient, should be constructed from assessment findings and should specify each rehabilitation problem identified, the program intervention selected to address that problem, and the expected outcome in measurable terms (see Table 3.1 for examples).

   D. Implementation forms: Flow sheets and/or progress notes designed to track the delivery of and responses to rehabilitation services

Implementation forms track the delivery of and responses to rehabilitation services.

      1. Flowsheets—for exercise, for education, for risk factor changes[1-6]

      2. Progress notes

         a. Content—status reports by rehabilitation staff members on patient performance in the program and progress to date toward rehabilitation goals

         b. Style—narrative commentary or subjective/objective assessment plan (SOAP) outline as compatible with staff experience and institution expectations

         c. Frequency—may vary from per-visit noting in high-risk participants to problem-oriented noting (noting only when problems occur) in those at low risk

      3. Progress letters—periodic (e.g., every month for Phase II, every 3 to 6 months for Phases III and IV) summaries of a participant's progress in the program, to be sent to patient, physician, and/or third party payor

   E. Evaluation forms

      1. Discharge plan—an outline of ongoing rehabilitation plans for the patient to follow after completion of the rehabilitation program

      2. Discharge summary—a synopsis of program results identifying exact outcomes achieved, commonly including linear and/or graphic comparisons of measurements taken before and after program participation and subjective surveys of patient satisfaction

      3. Completion of rehabilitation plan—documentation of extent of outcome achievement

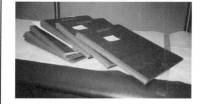

## Maintenance Program

The low-risk nature of patients stratified to maintenance programs and the community location of most maintenance programs enable more simplified participant record keeping than that outlined for post-hospital programs. The same medicolegal forms are required, but other intake information tends to be abbreviated. A plan still needs to be developed and outcomes projected. Typically, participants keep their own exercise records, which are reviewed and discussed with rehabilitation staff, who periodically prepare progress summaries.

## References

The following is a list of selected textbooks with sample forms and suggestions for cardiac rehabilitation documentation:

1. Comoss PM, Burke EAS, Swails SH. *Cardiac Rehabilitation: A Comprehensive Nursing Approach*. Philadelphia: JB Lippincott; 1979.
2. Franklin BA, Gordon S, Timmis GC. *Exercise in Modern Medicine*. Baltimore: Williams and Wilkins; 1989.
3. Hall LK, Meyer GC, Hellerstein HK. *Cardiac Rehabilitation: Exercise Testing and Prescription*. New York: Spectrum Publications; 1984.
4. Pashkow F, Pashkow P, Schafer M. *Successful Cardiac Rehabilitation*. Loveland, CO: HeartWatchers Press; 1987.
5. Pollock ML, Schmidt DH. *Heart Disease and Rehabilitation*. 2nd ed. New York: John Wiley and Sons; 1986.
6. Wilson PK, Fardy PS, Froelicher VF. *Cardiac Rehabilitation, Adult Fitness, and Exercise Testing*. 2nd ed. Philadelphia: Lea & Febiger; 1988.

# Chapter 7

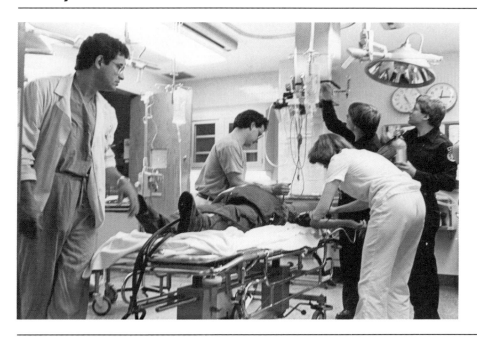

# Management of Emergencies

One of the major responsibilities of any cardiovascular or pulmonary rehabilitation program is to offer safe and efficacious treatment.[1-6] These treatments may include clinical laboratory analysis, graded exercise testing, metabolic studies, and supervised exercise therapy. Such services can, in rare instances, be associated with medical emergencies requiring immediate action. In addition, participants seen in these types of programs may exhibit early warning signs or symptoms of potential medical emergencies that would also require prompt intervention. The purpose of this section is to

- define staff training and certification in emergency cardiac care,
- describe certain early warning signs and symptoms of increasing risk that may require immediate medical intervention,
- discuss appropriate interventions,
- list emergency equipment necessary for participant safety, and
- provide guidelines for documentation and follow-up of emergency situations.

**Some cardiac rehabilitation services can, in rare instances, be associated with medical emergencies.**

## Training and Certification

The recommended training and certification programs for emergency cardiac care are those provided by the American Heart Association (AHA). It is recommended that *all staff* who relate to patient care, either in exercise, education, or administration, be certified in Basic Life Support (BLS) as designated by the AHA. It is also recommended that *all staff* (nonphysician) who are medically responsible for patients during dynamic activities (i.e., personnel who have been specifically designated by the medical director as having a direct medical role in the emergency plan) be certified in Advanced Cardiac Life Support (ACLS) as designated by the AHA. It is further recommended that one medical supervising staff who is both certified and licensed to provide ACLS be present during all dynamic activities. ACLS certification "does not warrant performance, nor does it, per se, qualify or authorize a person to perform any procedure. It is in no way related to licensure, which is a function of the appropriate legislative, health, or educational authority."[1] Licensure implies that personnel are licensed by their state to start intravenous therapy, deliver intravenous medication, and perform defibrillation. Certification in ACLS *does not license* an individual to perform these tasks. It is the responsibility of each program to have appropriately certified, licensed, and designated personnel to provide emergency cardiac care, including ACLS or Pediatric Advanced Life Support (PALS),[1,6] a new certification jointly sponsored by the American Academy of Pediatrics and the AHA. The latter would be appropriate for those centers testing and training pediatric patients, including those recovering from transplants and other major surgical procedures.

Community standards of care will direct each program in its personnel choice. The medical director of the program, or medical advisory committee, should be responsible for this designation. Regularly scheduled documented emergency "mock" codes should be held for all staff related to patient care. Regularly scheduled review of emergency cart equipment, medications, and supplies should be performed and documented. All staff who have direct or supervisorial contact with patients should participate in these mock codes and review of emergency medications, equipment, and supplies. A final and essential requirement is the writing and issuance of standing orders for emergency situations and full-blown codes. These should be posted and can rely heavily on ACLS-PALS guidelines. (See Forms A, B, and C in Appendix A.)

## Early Warning Signs and Symptoms of Increasing Risk

Changing patterns of signs or symptoms in clinical status can alert the rehabilitation staff to early warning signals that may precede cardiovascular complications and medical emergencies. These may include but are not limited to the following:

- Changing patterns of angina: The type, intensity, frequency, or duration of angina in patients with this symptom should be monitored regularly. If a patient reports that his or her customary treatment for angina is less effective than usual, this may signify a changing pattern of angina. Any report of at-rest or spontaneously

**One medical supervising staff person who is both certified and licensed to provide ACLS must be present during all dynamic activities.**

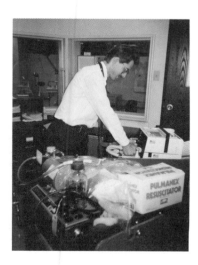

occurring angina should be conveyed to the patient's physician immediately. Patients should be educated in describing and defining their usual anginal symptoms in order to evaluate changing patterns. (See Form D.)

- New onset of angina in any patient should be immediately reported to the patient's referring physician.
- Arrhythmias: A changing pattern in the frequency, duration, or type of usual arrhythmia, especially any episodes of arrhythmia associated with lightheadedness. Patients should be educated in describing and defining their usual arrhythmias (e.g., via palpation) in order to evaluate changing patterns. (See Form E.)
- New onset of atrial or ventricular arrhythmias.
- Syncope or presyncope, especially if associated with arrhythmias.
- Symptoms of transient ischemic attack (TIA) or stroke.
- Symptoms of intermittent claudication.
- Indications of left ventricular (LV) dysfunction or congestive heart failure:
  - A change in the rating of perceived exertion with usual exercise, worsening or changing patterns of shortness of breath with exercise or at rest, or swelling of both ankles associated with weight gain.
  - Changing patterns of fatigue: increased fatigue with usual exercise patterns or the inability to sleep at night following normal exercise routines.

All indications of early warning signs and symptoms should be documented in the participant's chart, reviewed with the participant, and reported to the referring physician. Follow-up should include notes verifying any interventions or changes in medical therapy. (See Form F.)

**All indications of early warning signs and symptoms should be documented, reviewed with the patient, and promptly reported to the referring physician.**

## Interventions

With warning situations and emergencies and for general purposes of participant evaluation, clinical measurements should be taken, which may include the following:

- Self-reported history from the participant, which describes the symptoms she or he is experiencing.
- Blood pressure.
- Heart rate.
- Electrocardiographic monitoring for ST-segment displacement or arrhythmias.
- Standard 12-lead electrocardiogram (ECG) for indication of a changing pattern compared to prior resting ECG (e.g., evidence of myocardial infarction, ischemia, heart block, etc.). It is necessary to have a standard resting 12-lead ECG on all patients available for comparative purposes.
- Assessment of heart and lungs by auscultation.

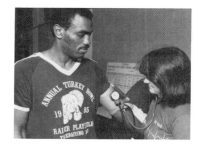

Interventions may include the following:

- Immediate phone call to the referring physician to report warning situation and receive orders

- The use of nitroglycerin
- The use of oxygen
- Establishment of intravenous fluids as a safety precaution or if a more complicated situation is anticipated
- Rapid transportation to closest emergency room
- ACLS as necessary

### In-Hospital Therapeutic Program

Appropriate surveillance of hospitalized patients, including ECG monitoring, clinical assessment, and other routine patient procedures to evaluate cardiovascular status and stability, should be performed and documented. These surveillance data should be a permanent written record in each participant's chart. Hospital-approved emergency guidelines should be updated regularly and adhered to. These guidelines must be written to cover all areas of the hospital where rehabilitation programs are held. Medications and equipment should be regularly reviewed, and this review documented. All policies and procedures should follow JCAHO regulations. Whenever possible, prior-to-discharge evaluation should include education regarding the reporting of early warning signs and symptoms to the appropriate medical personnel.

### Ambulatory and Outpatient Therapeutic Program

**All participants should be informed of early warning signs that may signify deterioration in their cardiovascular status.**

Information with regard to type of surveillance and emergency cardiac care that is available in the outpatient setting should be provided to all participants/patients. They should also be informed of early warning signs that may signify deterioration in their cardiovascular status. Outpatient therapeutic programs should provide a written record of each participant's symptoms or status by recording certain variables at each session, such as heart rate, angina, atrial and ventricular arrhythmias, blood pressure, medication changes, and orthopedic problems. Abnormal signs and symptoms should be discussed by the staff on a regular basis. There should be a method by which patients report, with each exercise therapy session, changes in medications. (See Form G.) Equipment capability and staffing to provide ACLS should be the same as described earlier. Clear descriptions of the emergency plans (e.g., paramedic response, code team response) and personnel qualifications in case of cardiovascular emergencies should be written and acknowledged as informed consent by the participant before entry into the exercise program. (See Form H.)

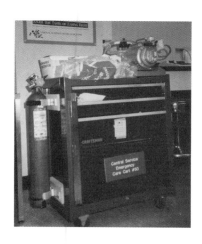

## Emergency Equipment

Emergency equipment should include, but is not necessarily limited to, the following:

- Portable battery-operated defibrillator with electrocardiographic printout and monitor, each with battery-low light indicator. DC capability in case of battery failure should be available for defibrillator, monitor, and ECG printout.
- Defibrillator with cardioversion and battery-check capability.

- Portable oxygen with nasal cannula, mouth-to-mouth, or bag-to-mouth unit with $O_2$ tubing.
- Portable suction equipment.
- Intravenous equipment with appropriate tubing and intravenous infusion fluid.
- ACLS medications as noted in AHA standards and based on community standard and medical advisory committee recommendations. (ACLS Drug Administration Schedule can be used as a basic unit.)
- Code phone, medical alert signal, or other emergency signal system to call for paramedics or code team as applicable.
- Intubation equipment available as appropriate to the program. If intubation equipment is available and planned to be used, personnel who are certified and licensed to perform intubation should be accessible to the program. (See ACLS guidelines.)
- Blood pressure measurement equipment. Anaeroid and mercury manometer are both recommended.
- Cart or appropriate storage unit for emergency equipment and medication. The emergency equipment and medication should be appropriately stored and secured out of reach of general public when not in use.
- All cardiovascular and pulmonary events must be clearly documented with outcome. This record must be made a permanent part of each patient's chart. A copy of this record should be sent to the referring physician.
- Biomedical engineering check of equipment for maintenance and performance every 6 months, or as JCAHO standards or state requirements apply. Documentation of such maintenance and a recording of the check should be performed as necessary and required.

### Exercise Testing Laboratory

Emergency and ergometric equipment should include, but is not necessarily limited to, the following:

- Multichannel ECG recorder with memory loop
- Examination table
- Treadmill with low-level capacity (e.g., 1.0 mph, 0% grade), calibrated on a regular basis
- Stationary cycle ergometer with accurate work-load indicator, calibrated on a regular basis
- Emergency drugs and equipment as listed previously under exercise therapy
- Biomedical engineering check of equipment for maintenance every 6 months, or as JCAHO standards or state requirements apply

## Documentation

The following is a list of forms found in Appendix A. In addition to the eight forms discussed in text, an Emergency Cart Checklist and a Mock Code Documentation form are included.

> All cardiovascular and pulmonary events must be clearly documented with outcome.

- Form A: Equipment for Adult Resuscitations
- Form B: Principles for the Management of Cardiac Arrest
- Form C: Sample Physician Standing Order
- Form D: Daily Log for Angina
- Form E: Daily Log for Arrhythmias
- Form F: Documentation of Emergency or Other Medical Intervention
- Form G: Exercise Therapy Record
- Form H: Informed Consent for Exercise Therapy
- Form I: Emergency Cart Checklist
- Form J: Mock Code Documentation

## References

1. American Heart Association. *Textbook of Advanced Cardiac Life Support*. Dallas, TX: AHA; 1987.
2. American Heart Association. *Textbook of Basic Life Support*. Dallas, TX: AHA; 1987.
3. American College of Sports Medicine. *Guidelines for Exercise Testing and Prescription*. Philadelphia: Lea & Febiger; 1986:23-24.
4. Fry G, Berra K. *YMCArdiac Therapy*. San Francisco, CA: Carolyn Bean & Associates; 1981.
5. North Carolina Department of Human Resources. *The Rules Governing the Certification of Cardiac Rehabilitation Programs*. Raleigh, NC: Division of Facility Services, Licensure and Certification Section. 1988.
6. American Heart Association. *Textbook of Pediatric Advanced Life Support*. Dallas, TX: AHA; 1988.

# Chapter 8

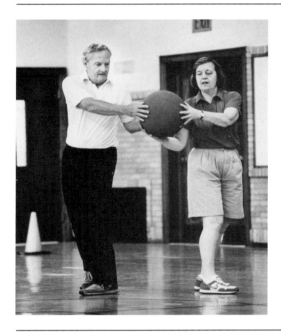

# Facilities and Equipment

Whatever the setting, the facilities and equipment used for providing cardiovascular and pulmonary rehabilitation must meet the requirements of federal, state, and local building safety codes.[1] They also must be adequate to meet the program's goals and objectives (as outlined in its Policy and Procedures Manual), with sufficient space available for the scope of services offered, including emergency care. A monitoring program of preventive maintenance and infection control should be documented and available for review, and equipment should be maintained and calibrated according to manufacturer recommendations.

## In-Hospital Phase

Convalescing cardiac patients are usually in an intensive care unit, surgical intensive care unit, intensive medical care unit, telemetry floor, step-down unit, or general medical floor. Therefore, cardiovascular and pulmonary rehabilitation services for in-hospital patients may occur at the bedside, in the hallway, or in a separate exercise or education location. Any of these areas must be in compliance with the JCAHO guidelines for patient safety.

Any area where cardiovascular or pulmonary rehabilitation services are provided must be in compliance with JCAHO guidelines.

The equipment utilized for in-hospital programs may vary widely. Most programs would require a form of ECG telemetry monitoring. This is usually a component of the nurse's station. Other types of equipment might include, but should not be limited to,

- stethoscope,
- portable sphygmomanometer, and
- other specific equipment needed to fulfill the requirements for exercise and education specific to the program scope of service (such as brochures, audiovisual tapes, pamphlets, and educational aids). Exercise supplies may include light weights, mild-resistance rubber bands, and sport balls.

In all cases, the educational materials required to fulfill discharge planning must be available. These would include the various components needed for educating the patient about risk factors, hygiene, sexuality, medications, and home programs.[2]

## Early Ambulatory Outpatient Therapeutic Program

**Exercise training can favorably modify several coronary risk factors.**

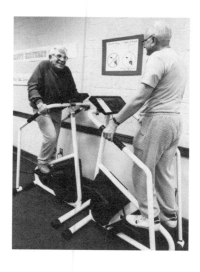

Exercise may be an effective intervention for the reduction of several coronary risk factors. Furthermore, exercise intervention is used to increase the patient's psychological well-being and functional capacity to enable a safe return to work and recreational and sexual activity. The use of exercise as an intervention in the rehabilitation of these patients involves specific facility and equipment requirements according to each patient's identified level of risk. In all cases, the facility should meet the standards as written elsewhere by the Joint Commission on Accreditation for Healthcare Organizations,[3] the American Heart Association,[4] and/or the American College of Sports Medicine.[5] The following list represents an example of equipment that may be used during the ambulatory therapeutic phase.

### Low-Risk Patients

*Lower extremity devices*
> Stationary bicycles, treadmills, stair-climbing device, walking area, and resistance equipment

*Upper extremity devices*
> Wall pulleys, dumbbells, rowing machines, arm ergometers, resistance equipment

*Combined upper and lower extremities*
> Cross-country ski machines, combined arm and leg ergometers, small-item equipment (such as wands, balls, rubber bands, resistive tubing, etc.), warm-up and cool-down area, general exercise area, and swimming pool

In all cases, the facility should meet the safety requirements to provide these services.

### Moderate-Risk Patients

Moderate-risk patients may be able to utilize all of the equipment mentioned above for the low-risk patient; however, it is advisable that ECG monitoring be available and employed in selected cases. Some patients may also use strength training devices, including free weights, and other types of resistive exercise equipment.

### High-Risk Patients

With the high-risk patient, it is highly recommended that ECG monitoring with printout be available and employed. Treadmills must be calibrated and provide a speed and elevation minimum that would fulfill the MET levels appropriate for the physical conditioning of such high-risk patients.

For all types of patients in the ambulatory therapeutic program, it is appropriate to have available the educational materials necessary to provide information about risk-factor modification. These materials would include scales, booklets, flip-charts, audiovisual aids, and any other references that would make the patient more aware of the disease process.

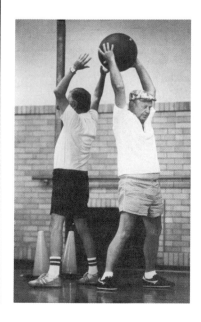

## Maintenance Program

The maintenance program is designed to provide continued support and supervision to the patient and family in an effort to continue the reduction of risk factors associated with the development of coronary artery disease. A variety of equipment and facilities can be used to achieve this goal. Depending upon the medical and functional status of the patient, such programs can be housed in YMCAs, Jewish community centers, shopping malls, hospital-based settings, and recreational and park areas of the community.

### Low-Risk Patients

Low-risk patients often are able to maintain their own exercise and education programs without a significant risk of complications. These patients may walk or jog on their own, join fitness facilities, or remain involved in wellness-type programs. In any case, the equipment and facilities used should be applicable for these patients as outlined earlier. If a facility does not have emergency equipment available, the patient should be informed (e.g., via a consent form).

### Moderate-Risk Patients

The moderate-risk patient may be more appropriately followed in a supervised program. The equipment and facilities for such programs should fulfill the written objectives in the Policy and Procedures Manual for the program. In all cases, emergency equipment should be available. The facility should allow for changing and showering areas. Equipment should provide sufficient workloads to enable a broad spectrum of patients to obtain a therapeutic range of exercise to improve or maintain their fitness levels. Educational materials may vary but should include information on how to prevent further complications. Often group facilities may include design modifications for volleyball, badminton, and other recreational activities that provide a psychosocial as well as an exercise rehabilitation component. If a pool is available and utilized by the program, it should have an appropriate area for group activities so that the patients can stand in the water while exercising. Appropriate water-safety equipment should be available as part of the requirements of the facility. The patients may also use buoys, kickboards, and other devices in such a program.

### High-Risk Patients

The high-risk patient in the maintenance program may benefit from periodic heart rate and rhythm checks, so it may be appropriate to have ECG readouts available from either a defibrillator or some type of monitoring ECG device. This equipment would be appropriate for low- and moderate-risk patients as well. The ability to quantitate work loads on the equipment is highly recommended so that MET levels appropriate to the functional capacity of the high-risk patient may be precisely regulated.

## Conclusion

In summary, cost effectiveness and patient outcomes need to be carefully balanced when one is making choices about the facilities and equipment required for effective cardiovascular and pulmonary rehabilitation. A number of programs throughout the country have provided appropriate facilities and equipment to several thousand patients to achieve desired patient outcomes. The key to the program is the staff understanding of the proper use of equipment and the layout of the facility. Regardless of the amount spent on equipment, proper use of it can facilitate an effective and safe patient outcome. To date, there have been no studies identifying the relative value of equipment in relation to cost and patient outcome. A variety of facilities and equipment are used with apparent effectiveness in helping patients reduce the risks and complications of cardiovascular and pulmonary disease.

Other types of equipment, including support-service apparatus such as desk, chairs, and filing cabinets, need to be given consideration. Appropriate supplies are always needed for programs to function effectively. Furthermore, it is strongly recommended that the medical records of the patients be protected for confidentiality and against fire and disaster.[6] These files should be locked at all times, when not in use, in a fire-resistant cabinet. Items such as electrodes, alcohol prep pads, and other such supplies should be stored in a sanitary and safe environment. Proper instruction in the use of such supplies should be provided by the therapists upon the initiation of the program.

Facilities and equipment are important at every stage of rehabilitation, but it is the staff's use of both that is paramount in providing safe and appropriate intervention programs for patients. If the resources of standards written elsewhere are used, the planning, operation, and ongoing activities of a program's facilities and equipment can fulfill the needs outlined in this section.

## References

1. Meyer GC. Organizational steps in initiating a cardiovascular rehabilitation program. In: Oldridge N, Foster C, Schmidt DH, eds.

**Cost effectiveness and patient outcomes need to be carefully balanced when making choices about facilities and equipment.**

**Facilities and equipment are important, but the staff's use of both is paramount.**

*Cardiac Rehabilitation and Clinical Exercise Programs: Theory and Practice.* Ithaca, NY: Mouvement Publications; 1988:314.
2. Miller MD. Health teaching in cardiac rehabilitation. In: Hall LK, Meyer GC, Hellerstein HK, eds. *Cardiac Rehabilitation: Exercise Testing and Prescription.* Champaign, IL: Human Kinetics; 1988:273-292.
3. Joint Commission on Accreditation of Healthcare Organizations. *Accreditation Manual for Hospitals,* Chicago, IL: Joint Commission on Accreditation of Healthcare Organizations; 1988.
4. The Committee on Exercise. *Exercise Testing and Training of Individuals with Heart Disease or at High Risk for Its Development: A Handbook for Physicians.* Dallas, TX: American Heart Association; 1975.
5. American College of Sports Medicine. *Resource Manual for Guidelines for Exercise Testing and Prescription.* Philadelphia: Lea & Febiger; 1988.
6. Department of Health and Human Services. *Health Care Financing Administration Part IV. Medicare Program; Comprehensive Outpatient Rehabilitation Facility Services; Final rule 47 (244) December 15, 1982.*

# Appendix A

# Sample Forms

**Form A**

## Equipment for Adult Resuscitations

Organize in sequence of use. A group may be placed in a clear bag, container, or specific area of a cart and sealed.

**A. Airway**

*Group 1: Initial*

Oral and nasal airways (large, medium, and small adult)

Face mask with one-way valve and oxygen inlet

$O_2$ connector to $O_2$ source and flow meter

$O_2$ tubing

*Group II: Secondary*

Tonsil tip and straight suction catheter

Wall outlet suction unit

Bag-valve-mask unit with $O_2$ reservoir

*Group III: Intubation*

Laryngoscope handle

Curved and straight adult blades

Endotracheal tubes and low-pressure cuffs, sizes 7, 8, 9

Stylet

Lubricating jelly and/or anesthetic jelly (water soluble)

10-mL syringe

Stethoscope

Optional

McGill forceps

Topical anesthetic spray

**B. Venous access**

*Group IV: Peripheral*

Alcohol or iodophor prep sponge

IV catheter (catheter-over-needle, 5-5.5 cm) 14 gauge (1 or more), 16 gauge (1 or more), 18 gauge (1 or more)

IV tubing—minidrip administration set (1 or more), stopcock (1 or more), IV extension set (1 or more)

5% dextrose/water 500 mL

2″ × 2″ sterile gauze sponges

1″ adhesive tape

Tourniquet

*Group V: Central*

Sterile drapes and gloves (masks, haircovers, sterile gown)

Iodophor prep solution

4″ × 4″ sterile gauze sponges

10-mL nonluerlock syringe

18-gauge, thin-wall, 6-cm-long needle

0.035 guidewire, at least 35 cm long

16-gauge 15- to 20-cm-long catheter

Suture material: 2-0 silk on curved needle, needle holder, scissors

IV tubing: minidrip administration set (1), stopcock (1), IV extension set (1)

5% dextrose/water 500 mL

Dressing material: iodophor or antibiotic ointment, gauze sponges, adhesive tape

**C. Additional equipment**

*Group VI: Equipment/fluids*

5% dextrose/water 250 mL (4)

5% dextrose/water 500 mL (2)

Normal saline 1,000 mL (2)

Lactate Ringer's 1,000 mL (2)

IV microdrip infusion pump tubing (4)

IV microdrip administration set (2)

IV maxidrip administration set (2)

IV extension set (2)

Blood administration set (2)

Blood pump

Armboard

Needles of various sizes—21 and 22 gauge, 3.5-4 cm; 22 gauge, 8.75 cm intracardiac

Syringes, various sizes, including one 50-mL glass syringe

Arterial blood gas sampling kits

16-gauge CVP catheter, 0.035 guidewire, 18-gauge thin-wall needle (2)

**(Cont.)**

## Form A (Continued)

16-gauge, 5-cm catheter-over-needle (4)
18-gauge, 5-cm catheter-over-needle (4)
Introducer sheath—8 French with high flow side arm (2)
Vascular cutdown tray
Alcohol or iodophor prep sponges
Iodophor or antibiotic ointment
Medication labels
Nasogastric intubation (all together in a plastic bag)
  Nasogastric tube
  Lubricating jelly
  Catheter tip syringe
  1″ tape
Additional endotracheal tubes, sizes 7, 8, 9
4″ × 4″ sterile gauze sponges

Sterile gloves, drapes, masks, haircovers, sterile gowns
Cardiac arrest board

**D. Optional equipment**
CVP manometer
Chest tubes
Chest drainage system, Heimlich valve
Emergency medication drug calculation sheets
$O_2$ cylinder and portable suction machine
External pacemaker
Percutaneous transvenous pacemaker
Transthoracic pacemaker
Pacemaker generator
Pericardiocentesis tray
Cricothyrotomy kit (scalpel and size 5 tracheostomy tube)

---

*Note.* Reproduced with permission. © *Textbook of Advanced Cardiac Life Support,* 1987. Copyright American Heart Association. (Material appears on p. 247.) A defibrillator may be used before the airway equipment.

# Principles for the Management of Cardiac Arrest

Many of these activities will be enacted simultaneously. Their order in this table does not mandate their exact sequence of occurrence in the code setting.

| Program | Equipment from cart | Intervention |
|---|---|---|
| 1. Recognition of arrest | | 1. Initiate CPR and call for help. |
| 2. Arrival of resuscitation team, emergency cart, monitor-defibrillator | 2. a. Cardiac board<br>b. Mouth-to-mask or bag-valve-mask unit with O₂ tubing<br>c. Oral airway<br>d. (Oxygen and regulator if not already at bedside) | 2. a. Place patient on cardiac board.<br>b. Ventilate with 100% $O_2$ with oral airway and mouth-to-mask or bag-valve-mask device.<br>c. Continue chest compressions. |
| 3. Identification of team leader | | 3. a. Assess patient.<br>b. Direct and supervise team members.<br>c. Solve problems.<br>d. Obtain patient history and information about events leading up to the code. |
| 4. Rhythm diagnosis | 4. Cardiac monitor with quick-look paddles–defibrillator (limb leads, ECG machine—12 lead) | 4. a. Apply quick-look paddles first.<br>b. Limb leads, but do not interrupt CPR. |
| 5. Prompt defibrillation if indicated | | 5. Use correct algorithm. |
| 6. Venous access | 6. a. Peripheral or central IV materials<br>b. IV tubing, infusion fluid | 6. a. Peripheral: antecubital.<br>b. Central: internal jugular, or subclavian. |
| 7. Drug administration | 7. Drugs as ordered (and in anticipation, based on algorithms) for bolus and continuous infusion | 7. a. Use correct algorithm.<br>b. Bolus or infusion. |
| 8. Intubation | 8. a. Suction equipment<br>b. Laryngoscope<br>c. Endotracheal tube and other intubation equipment<br>d. Stethoscope | 8. a. Connect suction equipment.<br>b. Intubate patient (interrupt CPR no more than 30 seconds).<br>c. Check tube position (listen for bilateral breath sounds). |
| 9. Ongoing assessment of the patient's response to therapy during resuscitation | | 9. Assess frequently:<br>a. Pulse generated with CPR (IS THERE A PULSE?);<br>b. Adequacy of artificial ventilation;<br>c. Spontaneous pulse after any intervention/rhythm change (IS THERE A PULSE?);<br>d. Spontaneous breathing with return of pulse (IS THERE BREATHING?);<br>e. Blood pressure, if pulse is present;<br>f. Decision to stop, if no response to therapy. |

**(Cont.)**

**Form B** **(Continued)**

| Program | Equipment from cart | Intervention |
|---|---|---|
| 10. Documentation | 10. Resuscitation record | 10. Accurately record events while resuscitation is in progress. |
| 11. Drawing arterial and venous blood specimens | 11. Arterial puncture and venipuncture equipment | 11. a. Draw specimens.<br>b. Treat as needed, based on results. |
| 12. Controlling or limiting crowd | | 12. Dismiss those not required for bedside tasks. |

*Note.* Reproduced with permission. ©*Textbook of Advanced Cardiac Life Support*, 1987. Copyright American Heart Association. (Material appears on p. 236.)

# Sample Physician Standing Order

Imprint patient's plate here.

| Time noted by nurse | | Ordered | | Diet, medication, treatment with doctor's signature |
|---|---|---|---|---|
| Hour | Name | Date | Hour | |
| | | | | Complete allergy information at time of admission. |
| | | | | Allergies: |
| | | | | CARDIAC ARREST: V. FIB OR PULSELESS V-TACH |
| | | | | ONE OR TWO STAFF PRESENT |
| | | | | WITNESSED VENTRICULAR FIBRILLATION OR PULSELESS |
| | | | | VENTRICULAR TACHYCARDIA |
| | | | | 1. Administer precordial thump |
| | | | | 2. Proceed with #2 below |
| | | | | UNWITNESSED VENTRICULAR FIBRILLATION OR PULSELESS |
| | | | | VENTRICULAR TACHYCARDIA |
| | | | | 1. Initiate CPR (Cardiopulmonary resuscitation) |
| | | | | 2. Initiate emergency protocol |
| | | | | 3. Verify cardiac rhythm and pulse |
| | | | | 4. Defibrillate at 200 joules |
| | | | | 5. Verify cardiac rhythm and pulse |
| | | | |    No pulse: Defibrillate at 200-300 joules |
| | | | | 6. Verify cardiac rhythm and pulse |
| | | | |    No pulse: Defibrillate at 360 joules |
| | | | | 7. No pulse: Continue CPR |
| | | | | MORE THAN TWO STAFF PRESENT |
| | | | | 8. Establish IV access |
| | | | | 9. Administer epinephrine 1:10,000 0.5-1.0 mg IVP |
| | | | |    (May be repeated at 5-minute intervals) |
| | | | | 10. Verify cardiac rhythm and pulse |
| | | | |    A. Defibrillate at 360 joules |
| | | | | 11. Administer lidocaine 1 mg/Kg IVP |
| | | | | 12. Continue to follow ACLS algorithms under |
| | | | |    medical supervision |
| | | | | |
| | | | | |
| | | | | |

_____          _____

(Supervising physician)                    (Medical department chair)     **(Cont.)**

**Form C (Continued)**

Imprint patient's plate here.

| Time noted by nurse | | Ordered | | Diet, medication, treatment with doctor's signature |
|---|---|---|---|---|
| Hour | Name | Date | Hour | |
| | | | | Complete allergy information at time of admission. |
| | | | | Allergies: |
| | | | | SUSTAINED VENTRICULAR TACHYCARDIA |
| | | | | |
| | | | | 1.  Recognition of sustained ventricular tachycardia |
| | | | | A.  Patient alert, awake, with pulse |
| | | | | 1.  Initiate emergency protocol |
| | | | | 2.  Apply $0_2$ via nasal cannula/face mask at 6 |
| | | | | L/min |
| | | | | MORE THAN TWO STAFF PRESENT: |
| | | | | 1.  Initiate IV access--give lidocaine bolus |
| | | | | 2.  Prepare for cardioversion |
| | | | | 3.  Continue to follow ACLS guidelines under medical |
| | | | | supervision |
| | | | | |
| | | | | |
| | | | | |
| | | | | |
| | | | | |
| | | | | |
| | | | | |
| | | | | |
| | | | | |
| | | | | |
| | | | | |
| | | | | |
| | | | | |
| | | | | |
| | | | | |
| | | | | |

_____           _____
(Supervising physician)                              (Medical department chair)

| Time noted by nurse | | Ordered | | Diet, medication, treatment with doctor's signature |
|---|---|---|---|---|
| Hour | Name | Date | Hour | |
| | | | | Complete allergy information at time of admission. |
| | | | | Allergies: |
| | | | | ABNORMAL RESPONSE |
| | | | | This includes a patient with new onset of chest |
| | | | | pain, shortness of breath (SOB), significant |
| | | | | hypotension, signs of ischemia, non-life-threatening |
| | | | | arrhythmias, or other indications of cardiac |
| | | | | compromise as determined by the cardiac staff |
| | | | | members. |
| | | | | |
| | | | | 1.  Identification of patient problem: |
| | | | | A.  Decrease or terminate exercise work load |
| | | | | B.  Assess heart rate and cardiac rhythm |
| | | | | C.  Assess blood pressure |
| | | | | 2.  Persistent anginal symptoms: |
| | | | | A.  Administer one (150 g) nitroglycerin tablet |
| | | | | SL |
| | | | | B.  Symptoms persist and blood pressure is |
| | | | | stable; repeat nitroglycerin in 5-minute |
| | | | | intervals two times (x's 2) |
| | | | | 3.  Unstable angina or new-onset angina: |
| | | | | A.  Apply $O_2$ at 2-6 L/min: nasal cannula/ |
| | | | | face mask |
| | | | | 4.  Monitor: Cardiac rhythm; heart rate; blood |
| | | | | pressure |
| | | | | |
| | | | | |
| | | | | |
| | | | | |
| | | | | |
| | | | | |

_____          _____

(Supervising physician)                    (Medical department chair)        **(Cont.)**

**Form C (Continued)**

| Time noted by nurse | | Ordered | | Diet, medication, treatment with doctor's signature |
|------|------|------|------|------|
| Hour | Name | Date | Hour | |
| | | | | Complete allergy information at time of admission. |
| | | | | Allergies: |
| | | | | ASYSTOLE |
| | | | | |
| | | | | 1. Recognition of asystole: verify in two leads |
| | | | | 2. Initiate CPR (Cardiopulmonary resuscitation) |
| | | | | 3. Initiate emergency protocol |
| | | | | MORE THAN TWO STAFF PRESENT |
| | | | | 4. Establish IV access |
| | | | | 5. Administer epinephrine 1:10,000 0.5-1.0 mg IVP |
| | | | | (May be repeated at 5-minute intervals) |
| | | | | 6. Check pulse |
| | | | | 7. NO PULSE: Administer atropine 1.0 mg IVP |
| | | | | (May repeat in 5 minutes x one [1]) |
| | | | | 8. Continue ACLS guidelines under medical |
| | | | | supervision |
| | | | | |
| | | | | |
| | | | | |
| | | | | |
| | | | | |
| | | | | |
| | | | | |
| | | | | |
| | | | | |
| | | | | |
| | | | | |
| | | | | |
| | | | | |
| | | | | |

_____     _____
(Supervising physician)                        (Medical department chair)

Imprint patient's plate here.

| Time noted by nurse | | Ordered | | Diet, medication, treatment with doctor's signature |
|---|---|---|---|---|
| Hour | Name | Date | Hour | |
| | | | | Complete allergy information at time of admission. |
| | | | | Allergies: |
| | | | | SYMPTOMATIC BRADYCARDIAC/SUPRAVENTRICULAR |
| | | | | TACHYCARDIA |
| | | | | |
| | | | | 1.  Recognition of patient problem: terminate |
| | | | |     exercise |
| | | | | 2.  Assess rhythm and blood pressure |
| | | | | 3.  Initiate emergency protocol |
| | | | | 4.  Apply $O_2$ nasal cannula/face mask at 4 L/min |
| | | | | 5.  Follow ACLS guidelines under medical supervision |
| | | | | |
| | | | | |
| | | | | |
| | | | | |
| | | | | |
| | | | | |
| | | | | |
| | | | | |
| | | | | |
| | | | | |
| | | | | |
| | | | | |
| | | | | |
| | | | | |
| | | | | |
| | | | | |
| | | | | |
| | | | | |
| | | | | |
| | | | | |

_____          _____
(Supervising physician)                          (Medical department chair)

# Daily Log for Angina

| # of Episodes | | | | | | | |
|---|---|---|---|---|---|---|---|
| Triggered | | | | | | | |
| Spontaneous | | | | | | | |
| Grade (1-4*) | | | | | | | |
| Duration | | | | | | | |
| Management | | | | | | | |
| Rest | | | | | | | |
| NTG | | | | | | | |
| Other | | | | | | | |

*Grade 1 is the onset of angina.
 Grade 4 is the worst angina you have experienced.

# Daily Log for Arrhythmias

| # of Episodes | | | | | | | |
|---|---|---|---|---|---|---|---|
| Trigger (if known) | | | | | | | |
| # Per minute | | | | | | | |
| Management | | | | | | | |
| Rest | | | | | | | |
| Medication | | | | | | | |
| Other | | | | | | | |

**Form F**

# Documentation of Emergency
# or Other Medical Intervention*

Patient name: _____ Date: _____

Summary of event:

Dispensation of patient:
(i.e., hospital/clinic/home)

Follow-up of outcome:

Date participant expected to return to program: _____

Staff signature: _____

*Attach appropriate physiological data such as 12-lead ECG, blood-pressure measurement, code form, etc., to this form.

All notes should be made a permanent part of the participant's record with appropriate incident form filled out as per usual community standard.

**Form G**

# Exercise Therapy Record

Participant name: _____ Date: _____

Heart rate prescription:

Heart rate with exercise today:

Exercise intervals/intensity today:

Blood pressure today:

Medication changes:

    1.

    2.

    3.

    etc.

Orthopedic problems:

    1.

    2.

    3.

    etc.

Other new/different medical concerns

# Informed Consent for Exercise Therapy

I desire to engage voluntarily in the _____
Cardiac Rehabilitation Program in order to improve my cardiovascular fitness. This program has been recommended to me by my physician, Dr. _____

Before I enter this program, I will have a clinical evaluation. This evaluation will include a medical history and physical examination consisting of but not limited to measurements of heart rate, blood pressure, and ECG at rest and with effort. The purpose of this evaluation is to detect any condition that would indicate that I should not engage in this exercise program.

The program will follow an exercise prescription prepared by _____
and will be carefully followed by the supervisor of the exercise program. The exercise prescription will be based upon my clinical evaluation. I agree to comply with the exercise prescription that I am given.

The activities that I will be given are designed to place a gradually increasing work load on the circulatory system and thereby improve its function. I understand that the reaction of the cardiovascular system to such activities cannot be predicted with complete accuracy. There is the risk of certain cardiovascular changes occurring during or following the exercise session. These changes may include abnormalities of blood pressure or heart rate, ineffective heart function, and, in rare instances, fatal or nonfatal heart attack or cardiac arrest.

Before starting the program I will be instructed as to the signs and symptoms that I should report promptly to the supervisor of the exercise session that would alert me to modify my activities. I understand that it is my responsibility to report to the staff any changes in my usual medications. I will report to the staff if I have to leave the exercise session early. I agree not to leave the exercise area without a cool-down period during which my heart rate has returned to its preexercise rate. Every effort will be made to avoid such events by clinical evaluation prior to beginning the exercise program and by observation during the exercise sessions. Emergency equipment and trained personnel are available to deal with and minimize the dangers of untoward events should they occur.

I have read the foregoing and I understand it. Any questions that have arisen or occurred to me have been answered to my satisfaction.

Date: _____

Participant signature: _____

Witness: _____

# Emergency Cart Checklist

## Daily Checklist

|  |  |  |  |  |  |  |  |  |  |  |  |  |  |  |  |  |  |  |
|---|---|---|---|---|---|---|---|---|---|---|---|---|---|---|---|---|---|---|
| 1. Defibrillator—discharges appropriate joules/amps |  |  |  |  |  |  |  |  |  |  |  |  |  |  |  |  |  |  |
| 2. Defibrillator battery registers full capacity |  |  |  |  |  |  |  |  |  |  |  |  |  |  |  |  |  |  |
| 3. Monitor displays accurate ECG per transmission of: paddles telemetry unit |  |  |  |  |  |  |  |  |  |  |  |  |  |  |  |  |  |  |
| 4. Monitor battery registers full capacity |  |  |  |  |  |  |  |  |  |  |  |  |  |  |  |  |  |  |
| 5. Electrocardiographic printout functions properly |  |  |  |  |  |  |  |  |  |  |  |  |  |  |  |  |  |  |
| 6. Electrocardiographic printout battery registers full capacity |  |  |  |  |  |  |  |  |  |  |  |  |  |  |  |  |  |  |
| 7. $O_2$ tank registers full capacity |  |  |  |  |  |  |  |  |  |  |  |  |  |  |  |  |  |  |
| 8. Suction machine functions with appropriate suction capacity |  |  |  |  |  |  |  |  |  |  |  |  |  |  |  |  |  |  |

## Monthly Checklist

| | | |
|---|---|---|
| 1. Medications: Name/dose/amount/expiration date For example: lidocaine/100 mg/3 vials/1.22.91 | | |
| 2. Intravenous supplies: Name/dose (if applicable)/amount/expiration date For example: dextrose 5% water/500 cc/3 units/1.15.91 | | |

# Maintenance and Calibration of Equipment

| | Date of most recent maintenance check | Date due for next maintenance check |
|---|---|---|
| 1. Defibrillator | | |
| Defibrillator batteries replaced | _____ | _____ |
| 2. Electrocardiographic monitor | _____ | _____ |
| 3. Electrocardiographic printout | _____ | _____ |
| 4. Oxygen tank | _____ | _____ |
| 5. Suction apparatus | _____ | _____ |

Maintenance problems noted:

1. _____

2. _____

3. _____

etc.

Program director notified (yes/no)

1. _____

2. _____

3. _____

etc.

# Mock Code Documentation

Date: _____

Staff at attendance:

    1.  _____

    2.  _____

    3.  _____

  etc. _____

| | | | | | | |
|---|---|---|---|---|---|---|
| Equipment drill | | | | | | |
| Defibrillation drill | | | | | | |
| Intravenous therapy review | | | | | | |
| Medication administration review | | | | | | |
| Transportation of participant review | | | | | | |
| Documentation of event review | | | | | | |

Staff ACLS/BLS certification:

Name: _____    Date due: _____

    1.  _____    _____

    2.  _____    _____

    3.  _____    _____

  etc. _____    _____

# Position Paper of the American Association of Cardiovascular and Pulmonary Rehabilitation

## Scientific Evidence of the Value of Cardiac Rehabilitation Services With Emphasis on Patients Following Myocardial Infarction

# Section 1

# Exercise Conditioning Component

**Arthur S. Leon, MD, Chairman;
Contributors: Catherine Certo, PhD, PT; Patricia Comoss, RN;
Barry A. Franklin, PhD; Victor Froelicher, MD;
William L. Haskell, PhD; Herman K. Hellerstein, MD;
William P. Marley, PhD; Michael L. Pollock, PhD; Andrew Ries, MD;
Erika Sivarajan Froelicher, PhD; L. Kent Smith, MD**

This position paper developed by an Ad Hoc Task Force of the American Association of Cardiovascular and Pulmonary Rehabilitation (AACVPR) assesses cardiac rehabilitation services in respect to objectives, components, phases, current requirements, patient benefits, mechanisms for observed benefits, effectiveness in reducing morbidity and mortality rates, and safety. The paper is divided into two sections. The focus in this section is on the exercise conditioning component and the next section is focused on the health education and risk factor and behavioral modification components.

## Purposes

Cardiac rehabilitative services originally were designed for patients recovering from an acute myocardial infarction (AMI). They subsequently have been expanded by modifying some of the procedures and therapeutic exercises to other coronary heart disease (CHD) patients including those recovering from coronary artery bypass graft surgery (CABGS) or percutaneous transluminal coronary angioplasty (PTCA), those with stable angina pectoris or silent ischemia, and as part of a primary prevention program for patients at high risk for a future CHD event due to their risk factor profile. These services also may be modified to meet the needs of patients with other forms of stable cardiac disease and uncomplicated cardiac surgical procedures, such as following heart valve replacement, correction of congenital heart defects, and heart transplantation.

The *ultimate* goal of cardiac rehabilitative services is to enable patients with cardiac disorders to resume active and productive lives within the limitations imposed by their disease process for as long as possible.[1] *Specific objectives* for accomplishing this goal include the following:[1-3]

1. Restoring individuals with cardiovascular disease to their optimal physiologic, psychosocial, and vocational status.
2. Prevention of progression or reversal of the underlying atherosclerosis process in patients with CHD or at high risk for CHD.
3. Reduction of risk of sudden death and reinfarction and alleviation of angina pectoris in CHD patients.

## Components

Medically supervised exercise conditioning is the focal point of cardiac rehabilitative programs and also what primarily differentiates them from simple counseling services.[4] Other essential elements include assessment of CHD patients for risk of future cardiovascular events and premature mortality, patient education, vocational guidance and risk factor modification (smoking cessation, weight management, lipid-lowering dietary and pharmacologic strategies, control of hypertension and diabetes, and stress management).

A multidisciplinary healthcare team is required to carry out this battery of services in cooperation with the patient's primary care physician. This

*Note.* This article is from the *Journal of Cardiopulmonary Rehabilitation,* 1990;10:79-87. Copyright 1990 by J.B. Lippincott Company. Adapted by permission.

team may include cardiologists or other physicians, nurses, psychologists or psychiatrists, nutritionists or dieticians, exercise physiologists, physical and occupational therapists, vocational counselors, health educators, and others. The program carried out by the rehabilitative team, by necessity, must be flexible and individualized since patients' medical problems and needs, educational level, and social and vocational situations vary a great deal.

## Phases

There are a number of ways of classifying the different phases of cardiac rehabilitation. Currently, cardiac rehabilitation services generally are divided into three or four phases—*Phase I*: the hospital inpatient period, ordinarily 6-14 days in length for patients with AMI or following CABGS; *Phase II*: the convalescent stage following hospital discharge (generally 8-12 weeks duration); *Phase III*: the supervised portion of the continued development/maintenance period (usually 4-6 months duration); *Phase IV*: the unsupervised portion of the ongoing maintenance period (indefinite in length). There are many excellent detailed descriptions available of sequential progressive arm and leg exercises, and principles of exercise prescription for cardiac patients commonly employed during each phase of a rehabilitation program and these will not be repeated here.[5-8] The health education, risk factor-behavior modification, and other supportive services are initiated for hospitalized patients during the in-hospital phase and are continued following hospital discharge.

An important recent addition to the rehabilitative process for the CHD patient initiated during Phase I or within a few weeks following hospital discharge is *risk stratification*, i.e., assessment of prognosis for future major CHD events and survival, particularly, during the first year following an AMI or CABGS. Various guidelines and algorithms have been proposed for risk stratification based on assessment of the extent of myocardial damage, left ventricular function, and presence or absence of residual myocardial ischemia and ventricular arrhythmias.[9,10] Noninvasive tools for these assessments include clinical variables during hospitalization for AMI, extent of QRS abnormalities on the resting ECG, low level exercise testing, resting and exercise radionuclide ventriculography or echocardiography, and 24-hour ambulatory ECG monitoring. Low-risk patients, who constitute be-

tween one third to one half of those following an AMI and about three quarters of patients who have undergone CABGS, have a first-year mortality rate of less than 2%.[9,10] In contrast, moderate-risk patients have a first-year mortality rate of 10% to 25% and high-risk patients greater than 25%. The results of this assessment process determine requirements for additional diagnostic and therapeutic procedures, possible contraindications to exercise training, the exercise prescription, and the degree of supervision required during an exercise program. Prognostically important abnormalities on the commonly performed predischarge, low level exercise test include ST segment depression, angina pectoris, inability to complete a low level of exercise (i.e., < 5 METs), inadequate systolic blood pressure response, and ventricular arrhythmias. Exercise test results are also useful for advising appropriate home activities and for designing a postdischarge exercise program.

Patients identified at increased risk for premature mortality are candidates for coronary arteriography and ventriculography to determine suitability for myocardial revascularization procedures. In contrast, low-risk patients require less intensive diagnostic and therapeutic interventions and have a greater potential for functional recovery and return to work soon after an AMI or CABGS.[9,10] Phase II convalescent programs usually commence as soon as possible after hospital discharge, although patients who have not been hospitalized may be referred to such programs. This phase usually is approximately 8-12 weeks duration; however, some patients may require 6 months or a year before achieving optimal functional improvement allowing independent maintenance of a desired style of life and activity. In Europe, Phase II programs are often carried out in special sanitariums.[11] In the United States, these physician-supervised programs usually are situated in either hospital outpatient facilities or community centers such as a YMCA or university gymnasium. All facilities must have available appropriate drugs, equipment and trained personnel for cardiopulmonary resuscitation and advanced life support and a physician in attendance or on call in the immediate vicinity in the advent of an emergency.[12]

Recent studies have demonstrated the feasibility and safety of prescriptive home exercise programs with intermittent transtelephonic ECG monitoring in selected low-risk convalescing CHD patients.[13] However, most authorities recommend exercise in a group setting, at least initially, during early convalescence because of a number of advantages over home exercise programs.[5] These advantages include the presence of healthcare personnel for exercise guidance, monitoring of heart rate, blood pressure, ECG, compliance with exercise prescription, and for emergency care in the advent of an exercise-induced complication. In addition, group programs offer greater opportunities for patient education and provide psychosocial support and companionship during exercise, which may help promote program compliance. Personal patient contact by a nurse or allied health professional also has been shown to improve compliance to preventive or rehabilitation program.[14,15]

Supervised Phase II exercise programs appear particularly useful for higher risk patients, for those who perform heavy physical labor on the job and/or vigorous recreational pursuits and for those who need reinforcement for health behavioral changes and risk factor modification.[1,4,16] Electrocardiogram monitoring, one of the traditional safety features of Phase II programs, has recently come under close scrutiny.[16,17] Intuitively, ECG telemetry during a supervised exercise program would appear to provide a "safety net" for cardiac patients by increasing the likelihood of detecting potentially serious arrhythmias and ischemic ST-segment changes and to assess compliance with heart rate prescriptions. Support for its routine use comes from a survey carried out over 10 years ago by Haskell.[18] A significantly lower cardiac event rate was found in the two programs out of 50 surveyed which employed continuous ECG monitoring; however, this observation was not substantiated by a more recent, larger scale survey by Van Camp and Peterson.[19] In the latter study, there were no significant differences in rates of cardiac arrest, recurrent myocardial infarctions, or fatalities during exercise between programs using continuous ECG monitoring versus those using either intermittent monitoring alone or initial continuous monitoring for at least three sessions followed by intermittent monitoring. Based on the above considerations and the fact that continuous monitoring adds substantially to the cost of a Phase II program, recent American College of Cardiology guidelines call for ECG monitoring only in moderate- or high-risk cardiac rehabilitation patients exhibiting significantly depressed left ventricular function, resting or exercise-induced complex ventricular arrhythmias, decreased systolic blood pressure during exercise, survivors of sudden death, complications following myocardial infarction, or if the patient is unable to self monitor exercise heart rate.[3] These criteria would be expected to eliminate the requirement of an extended period of ECG monitoring for about 75%-80% of AMI patients in Phase II rehabilitation programs.[3] Additional research is required to more adequately define the need for and the optimal duration of ECG monitoring. In the interim, it appears prudent to provide differing degrees of ECG monitoring based on the patient's clinical status, functional capacity, and prognosis following triage and risk stratification.

Another area which has generated controversy, is the role of arm exercise, particularly static (isometric) strength training, in a cardiac rehabilitation program. In the past, these forms of exercise were prohibited for cardiac patients because of concerns about possible adverse hemodynamic effects. However, recent studies have demonstrated the feasibility and effectiveness in improving arm strength and the safety of arm exercise training in selected CHD patients.[20] The prevalence of arrhythmias or other signs or symptoms during upper extremity training is reported to be no greater than during lower extremity training.[21-23] These findings are particularly relevant to patients who require a high level of upper body muscular strength for their preferred vocational and recreational activities. In addition many activities of daily living require static arm work.

A symptom-limited, graded exercise test usually is performed between the third and sixth week of a Phase II program. The results of this test are useful for adjusting the patient's exercise prescription, for evaluating the need for continued ECG monitoring during the exercise program, and to assess the adequacy of the patient's physical capacity to return to work. An exercise capacity of 9 METs or more without significant cardiac symptoms or signs is believed to be sufficient to allow more cardiac patients to return to jobs requiring light to moderate physical exertion or be triaged into a home or non-ECG monitored, supervised program.[16] Significant cardiac abnormalities on this exercise test indicate the need for further cardiac evaluation and treatment as well as for medical supervision and ECG monitoring during exercise conditioning.

Phase III maintenance exercise programs generally are based in a community recreational facility. Cardiac patients enrolled in community exercise program settings ideally should have successfully progressed through inpatient and convalescent exercise programs; however, low-risk cardiac patients with good functional capacity may be directly referred to a Phase III program without previous exercise program participation. As a general rule, cardiac patients in such programs should be at least 6-12 weeks posthospitalization, and clinically stable with a minimal functional capacity of 5 METs.[4] Patients generally remain in such a program for at least 4-6 months, during which time efforts are made to gradually reduce supervision and to promote self regulation of their exercise programs, hopefully for life. Exercise testing and medical evaluation should be repeated every 3-6 months during Phase III and eventually on an annual basis or as indicated clinically.[5] The patient's physician may refer him/her back to a medically supervised program if there is symptomatic deterioration, compliance problems, recurrence of angina pectoris, reinfarction, CABGS, or coronary angioplasty.

# Estimated Requirements for Rehabilitation Services

Coronary heart disease, the major reason for referral for cardiac rehabilitation services, is estimated to afflict 5.7 million Americans.[1] About one-quarter of this CHD population has stable angina pectoris. The annual incidence of AMI in the United States is about 1.5 million with about one third of the events representing reinfarction. About one out of every four or five patients with AMI expire prior to arrival at an acute care facility or shortly following hospitalization, usually within 2 hours of the onset of symptoms, due to a cardiac arrhythmia or pump failure. It is estimated that about two thirds of AMI survivors or approximately 500,000 people a year have no contraindications for admission to an exercise program. Another major potential source of clients for rehabilitation services are patients undergoing revascularization procedures, including the over 200,000 patients per year undergoing CABGS and over 200,000 per year following PTCA. Currently it is estimated that only about 100,000 persons per year in the United States are actually taking advantage of comprehensive cardiac rehabilitation programs, which represents about 11% of the CHD patient population. Patients with other forms of heart disease or cardiac surgical procedures are other potential candidates for cardiac rehabilitation services.

# Benefits of Exercise Training

## Counteracting Effects of Inactivity

The value of early mobilization and progressive ambulation and exercise for patients with AMI or following cardiac surgical procedures in counteracting the deleterious physiological effects of bed rest is well documented.[24,25] These deleterious effects include reduced physical work capacity, moderate tachycardia, skeletal muscle wasting with loss of strength, reduced pulmonary function, loss of postural vasomotor reflexes resulting in orthostatic hypotension, decreased circulatory blood volume, and increased risk of thromboembolism.

## Improved Functional Capacity

Another important contributor to reduced physical work capacity and maximal oxygen uptake ($\dot{V}O_2$max) level in patients following an AMI is a reduction in maximal cardiac output. This is primarily due to a decrease in maximal stroke volume related to the extent of myocardial damage.[26,27] Ischemia induced during physical exertion, with or without accompanying angina pectoris, also may contribute to reduced functional capacity. Such ischemia generally occurs at a reproducible threshold indicated by the product of heart rate and systolic blood pressure, a major determinant of myocardial oxygen requirements.[26,28]

Coronary heart disease patients typically show a substantial improvement in $\dot{V}O_2$max during cardiac rehabilitation. The increase in $\dot{V}O_2$max in AMI patients ranges from 11% to 56% and in CABG patients from 14% to 66% after 3-6 months of exercise training.[8,26,27] The greatest improvement can be expected in those patients with the lowest initial $\dot{V}O_2$max level. A major part of this improvement in patients following an AMI is due to the natural process of recovery and resumption of usual routine physical activities.[1,9,29] The additional increase in $\dot{V}O_2$max and physical work capacity induced by training for most CHD patients is predominately a result of peripheral adaptations, resulting in an increase in oxygen extraction and utilization by active skeletal muscle and an associated increase in arteriovenous oxygen difference.[1,26,27,30] However, it has recently been demonstrated by Ehsani et al.[31] that central myocardial adaptations by endurance exercise training in selected CHD patients also may contribute to increased $\dot{V}O_2$max similar to effects in healthy adults. These investigators found that prolonged (1 year or more), intense exercise training (85% or more of the maximal heart rate reserve) in patients after an AMI can substantially improve left ventricular contractile function as evidenced by an increase in ejection fraction, stroke volume, and rate pressure product (RPP) during maximal exercise. It should be noted that a vigorous training regime, such as employed by Ehsani et al.[31] is only appropriate for carefully selected cardiac patients because of the potential of precipitating a major coronary event.

## Improved Cardiovascular Efficiency

Although the improvement of maximal work capacity is the usual expressed physiologic goal of endurance exercise training, the CHD patient seldom has any direct need for the acquired increased capability for peak performance. The principal advantage for most CHD patients from a higher $\dot{V}O_2$max level is instead an increased tolerance for daily life activities consisting of repeated submaximal physical exertion. Submaximal effort after training can be accomplished at a lower percentage of $\dot{V}O_2$max resulting in greater endurance and less fatigue. In addition, heart rate, systolic blood pressure, and RPP are generally lower during submaximal efforts after exercise conditioning reducing myocardial oxygen demands.[26,30] These latter adaptations are particularly important to the CHD patient with exertional ischemia, especially those with accompanying angina pectoris. Exercise tolerance is generally increased with exercise conditioning in patients with stable angina pectoris because of a reduction in myocardial oxygen demands at the intensity of external work which produced ischemia prior to training. Reported improvements in symptom-limited $\dot{V}O_2$max in patients with angina pectoris range from 32% to 56%.[26]

## Possible Increase in Myocardial Vascularity

Exercise training in a number of animal species has been shown to increase myocardial vascularity, including augmentation of capillary density and enlargement of luminal areas of main and collateral coronary arteries.[32-35] Of particular relevance to the CHD patient is the finding by Kramsch et al.[34] that monkeys on atherogenic diets that jogged three times a week on motorized treadmills developed substantially larger coronary luminal areas and less severe coronary atherosclerosis as compared to sedentary control animals. Experiments in intact dogs and pigs also have demonstrated that exercise training potentiates the development of coronary collateral arteries induced by chronic narrowing or gradual occlusion of a major coronary artery.[32,33,35] However, there is limited confirmatory data in humans with or without CHD that exercise improves myocardial vascularity.

Rose et al.[36] at autopsy found significantly larger coronary arteries in men who had performed heavy physical labor as compared to less active workers. Those with larger coronary artery size also were less likely to have evidence of myocardial infarction. Coronary arteriography has proven useful for accurately delineating coronary collateral vessel size during life. This technique has confirmed postmortem and animal experimental observations that coronary artery stenosis and associated myocardial ischemia are potent stimuli for promoting coronary collateral formation.[32] There have been only a few isolated demonstrations by serial coronary arteriography of increased collateral development in CHD patients on exercise programs.[1,32,37,38] For example, Ferguson et al.[37] reported increased collateralization in only 4 of 14 CHD patients and Connor et al.[38] in two of six CHD patients after 10-13 months of supervised exercise training. In both of these studies it was suggested that the observed increases in coronary collateral development may have reflected a worsening of severity of coronary artery disease rather than the beneficial effects of exercise.

There is indirect supporting evidence that exercise conditioning can increase maximal myocardial blood flow and oxygen supply. A higher RPP prior to development of angina[26,32,39,40] and regression of ECG evidence of ischemia (ST segment displacement) at the same or a higher RPP has been reported in CHD patients in some, but not all, studies.[31,41] In addition, Froelicher et al.[42-44] reported an improvement in the mean thallium-201 myocardial scintigraphy ischemia score in a heterogenous group of CHD patients after 1 year of exercise training. Surprisingly, however, this was not accompanied by reduction in exercise-induced ischemia ST segment depression.[44] Thus, from the available human data it would appear that an exercise program in a CHD patient can improve myocardial profusion as well as reduce myocardial oxygen demands.

## Reduction of Risk Factors for CHD

Another well-documented potential benefit of an endurance exercise conditioning program is its favorable impact on major risk factors for atherosclerosis and CHD as demonstrated predominately in studies involving healthy volunteers. This topic was reviewed elsewhere.[45] Risk factors favorably altered by exercise training include loss of excess weight,[46] an increase in high density lipoproteins (HDL) cholesterol levels,[47] a reduction in elevated blood pressure levels,[48] and improvement in glucose–insulin dynamics.[49] These adaptations theoretically should contribute to the rehabilitative objective of slowing progression of atherosclerosis or perhaps even reversing its severity in CHD patients, although this remains to be proven.

## Possible Improvement in Psychological Well-Being

Another common rationale for exercise training of patients with CHD is to improve psychosocial functioning. There is a common perception among health professionals and among people who exercise regularly that exercise produces psychological benefits, including reducing anxiety, muscular tension and depression, and promoting a feeling of well-being.[50,51] However, most of the encouraging reports of the psychological benefits of exercise, particularly in cardiac patients, are based on clinical impression, anecdotal in nature, or attributed to studies which have major methodological problems. Methodological problems include small sample size, absence of a nonexercise control group, nonrandom design, inappropriate measures of psychological constructs, and investigator or subject bias.[50-52] A review of over 1000 articles on the psychological effects of exercise conditioning by Hughes[51] revealed only 12 which met the criteria for well-designed scientific studies. Furthermore, none of these controlled studies revealed significantly improved psychological functioning with exercise training, except for improved self-concept. Negative studies included the National Exercise and Heart Disease Project,[53] which involved 651 Americans with recent AMI randomly assigned to either an intense exercise group or a control group after an initial period of low intensity exercise for all subjects. In a more recent, well controlled, smaller scale study, Blumenthal et al.[52] compared the psychological effects of 12 weeks of moderate to high intensity vs low intensity exercise training in patients with recent AMI. No differences were found between groups in any measures of psychosocial functioning, including anxiety, depression, stress, and type A behavior. Based on these findings it was concluded that there is in-

adequate scientific evidence to support the role of exercise for improving the psychological well-being of the cardiac patient.[16,52] Blumenthal et al.[52] instead felt that a more direct approach, such as stress management or group therapy, may be more effective than exercise in reducing psychological dysfunction sometimes accompanying AMI or other cardiac disorders.

## Secondary Prevention of CHD Events

The evidence is inconclusive as to whether or not regular exercise reduces the possibility of recurrence of AMI, other clinical manifestations of CHD, and associated premature mortality. Supporting evidence for this hypothesis comes from observational epidemiological studies. These studies suggest that regular physical activity plays an important role in reducing risk of initial CHD events and mortality even in middle-aged men at high risk for CHD because of a combination of elevated levels of blood cholesterol, blood pressure, and cigarette smoking.[54-56] An inverse association also has been reported between physical fitness level and risk of initial CHD events.[57,58]

It has been estimated that a definitive randomized, controlled clinical trial to test the hypothesis that exercise reduces subsequent morbidity and from CHD mortality would require at least 4200 patients with recent AMI to be studied over a 5–7 year follow-up period.[59] To date none of the reported randomized secondary CHD trials to test the *independent* effect of exercise have had sufficient number of patients and/or were of sufficient duration to provide adequate statistical power to demonstrate the possible protective effect of exercise. It also appears unlikely that a definitive multicenter exercise secondary prevention trial of the required magnitude will ever be undertaken. This is because of major logistical problems including finding sufficient patients willing to be randomized, compliance issues (large dropout and crossover rates), the confounding effect of alterations in other CHD risk factors, the relatively low CHD recurrence rate among qualified low risk volunteers, the high financial costs, and other difficult issues. However, most of the reported randomized secondary prevention trials have demonstrated a favorable trend for a lower mortality rate in the exercise group as compared to the control group. For example, in the National Exercise and Heart Disease Project, a 3-year controlled, randomized trial in the United States on the effects of prescribed supervised exercise involving 651 men with AMI, the cumulative 3-year total mortality rate was 7.3% for the control group and 4.6% for the exercise group while the rate for recurrent MI was 7.0% and 5.3%, for the control and exercise group respectively.[59] It was estimated that if these trends favoring the exercise group had continued they would have reached statistical significance if 1500 patients had been enrolled in the study. On the other hand, in another large-scale North American study, the Ontario Heart Study,[60] in which 633 patients were followed for 4 years, trends for recurrence of both fatal and nonfatal MI were in favor of the control group, which was on a program of light exercise.

Two clinical trials in Europe with favorable outcomes randomized patients following an MI to either a multifaceted risk factor intervention–health education program, including exercise, or a control group. One of these studies, which involved fewer than 100 patients, found that a 6-week rehabilitation program was associated with a 50% lower rate of combined CHD morbidity (including occurrence of severe angina pectoris) and mortality in the "rehabilitated" as compared to the control patients over a 5-year follow-up period.[61] The second of these comprehensive multiple risk factor intervention studies involved 375 consecutive men and women AMI patients below 65 years of age in two clinical centers in Finland.[62] After 3 years of follow-up the cumulative CHD mortality rate was significantly smaller in the intervention group as compared to the control group (18.6% versus 29.4%) primarily due to a reduction in sudden death in the intervention group during the first 6 months after AMI. There also was a favorable trend towards reduction in nonfatal reinfarctions in the intervention group. It should be pointed out that mean exercise capacities as measured by cycle ergometer were similar in both groups at 1, 2, and 3 years of follow-up, indicating that the exercise program in this study was not of a strenuous nature. In addition, there were significantly greater reductions in levels of serum cholesterol, triglycerides, and systolic and diastolic blood pressure in the intervention group as compared to the control group.

An alternate but less rigorous scientific approach, in lieu of a definitive clinical trial, has been to pool data from existing long-term, randomized, secondary prevention trials in which exercise training was included. A number of these meta-analyses have been published in which data from 6 to 22 randomized long-term clinical trials were

pooled using the intention-to-treat principle.[59,63-66] In most of the trials included in these analyses, intervention consisted of an exercise program or exercise advice in combination with risk factor management making it impossible to "tease out" the independent contribution of exercise to subsequent morbidity and mortality. However, these meta-analyses revealed that patients randomized to comprehensive cardiac rehabilitation programs following an AMI had statistically significant reductions of at least 25% in 1- to 3-year rates of fatal cardiovascular events and in rate of total mortality as compared to control patients; however, no significant differences were found in rate of nonfatal recurrent reinfarctions in patients undergoing intervention as compared to control patients. It is of interest that the reduction in mortality attributed to cardiac rehabilitation indicated by these pooled data is similar in extent to the salvage rate attributed to beta blocking drugs in clinical trials following an AMI.[63]

There currently are no morbidity and mortality data from controlled clinical trials available showing the effects of cardiac rehabilitation programs on patients with stable angina pectoris or following CABGS or PTCA. Progression of atherosclerosis and closure of CABGS grafts and vessels undergoing coronary angioplasty remain problems following these procedures. It is hoped that a comprehensive rehabilitation program including multiple risk factor intervention and exercise training will prove to be helpful in secondary prevention following these revascularization procedures, but this also remains to be proven.

## Safety

Cardiac complications during cardiac rehabilitation programs include cardiac arrest, cardiac arrhythmias requiring cardioversion, AMI, pulmonary embolism, pulmonary edema, cardiogenic shock, unstable angina, and syncope.[18,19,27] Cardiac arrest is the most common of these complications and is seven times more frequent than the second most common recurrent nonfatal MI. The most comprehensive study of the incidence of such cardiovascular complications during rehabilitation recently was reported by Van Camp Peterson.[19] This survey was based on data obtained from 167 randomly selected programs from throughout the United States involving 51,303 patients, who exercised a total of over 2 million hours during the period

1980–1984. Twenty-one cardiac arrests (18 successfully resuscitated and 3 fatal) and eight nonfatal AMI were reported. The rate of complications were one cardiac arrest per 111,996 hours, one AMI per 293,900 hours and one fatality per 783,976 hours of prescribed supervised exercise. This relatively high level of safety was attributed to proper patient evaluations, education, and treatment; careful exercise prescription; appropriate degrees of ECG monitoring; well-trained personnel; and rapid, effective handling of emergencies. These data also suggest an improvement in the cardiac complication rates as compared to an earlier survey by Haskell[18] involving 30 cardiac rehabilitation centers and reports from individual rehabilitation centers.[67,68] In Haskell's survey one cardiac arrest was reported for every 33,000 hours of patient rehabilitation activity and one death for every 120,000 patient hours. The apparent safety of home exercise programs in selected CHD patients was previously referred to.[13]

## Summary and Conclusions

Medically prescribed and supervised exercise as part of a comprehensive rehabilitation program is a well-accepted standard for care throughout the world for cardiac patients, particularly following an acute myocardial infarction or coronary revascularization procedure. Early exercise testing for such patients is now considered an essential component of such a program for risk stratification to identify those needing additional diagnostic procedures and therapeutic care and for prescribing appropriate physical activity. Once patient risk is determined only moderate to high risk patients should be continued on daily telemetric ECG monitoring. There is substantial evidence that a minimum of 2–3 months and ideally at least 6 months of medically supervised exercise conditioning will result in cardiovascular adaptations which will optimize functional capacity and help the patient to resume an active, productive life. It is hoped that this period also will provide reinforcement to motivate the patient to continue physical conditioning and modification of other risk factors for life. However, this has not been scientifically documented.

Well-documented physiological adaptations from the conditioning program include peripheral changes involving the active skeletal muscle. These changes are the principal contributors to demonstrated increases in maximal aerobic capacity, endurance, and muscular strength. High intensity, longer term exercise programs also may favorably improve myocardial function in selected cardiac patients. Although experimental animal work suggests that myocardial vascular supply may also be augmented by endurance exercise training, this has not been adequately confirmed in patients with coronary heart disease. Instead, a reduction in myocardial oxygen demands through lowering of heart rate and systolic blood pressure during submaximal physical exertion is more likely to contribute to a restoration in the balance between myocardial oxygen on supply and demand in patients with underlying ischemia.

There also is substantial experimental evidence that endurance exercise conditioning can favorably alter several other risk factors for coronary heart disease. This theoretically should have a favorable impact on the underlying atherosclerotic process, but it remains to be proven.

Although it is generally assumed by both health professionals and exercisers that exercise conditioning promotes psychosocial well-being, it has not as yet been possible to demonstrate this by controlled studies.

There also has not been a definitive randomized clinical trial on the independent effect of exercise in prevention of recurrent coronary events in patients recovering from myocardial infarction, coronary bypass graft surgery, or angina pectoris. Pooling of data from existing controlled randomized trials involving patients recovering from an acute myocardial infarction provides supportive evidence that a comprehensive cardiac rehabilitation program can reduce premature mortality from cardiovascular events in such patients, but probably not nonfatal reinfarctions. The risk of major cardiovascular events and fatality associated with supervised cardiac rehabilitation programs appears to be quite low.

It is concluded that there is sufficient existing evidence supporting the importance of exercise in the rehabilitation of the cardiac patient even though vigorous scientific proof is still lacking to document all of the postulated benefits.

## References

1. National Center for Health Services Research and Health Care Technology Assessment. *Health Technology Assessment Reports. Cardiac*

*Rehabilitation Services*. Rockville, MD: U.S. Dept. of Health and Human Services; 1957: 1-89. DHHS Publication No (PHS) 88-3427.

2. Hellerstein HK, Ford AB. Rehabilitation of the cardiac patient. *JAMA*. 1957;164:225-231.

3. Recommendations of the American College of Cardiology on cardiovascular rehabilitation. *J Am Coll Cardiol*. 1986;7:451-453.

4. Health and Public Policy Committee, American College of Physicians. Cardiac rehabilitative services. *Ann Intern Med*. 1988;1098:671-673.

5. American College of Sports Medicine. *Guidelines for Exercise Testing and Prescription*. 3rd ed. Philadelphia: Lea & Febiger; 1986:53-71.

6. Wenger NK, Hellerstein HK. *Rehabilitation of the Coronary Patient*. 2nd ed. New York: John Wiley & Sons; 1984:197-284.

7. Fardy PS, Yankowitz FG, Wilson PK. *Cardiac Rehabilitation, Adult Fitness, and Exercise Testing*. 2nd ed. Philadelphia: Lea & Febiger; 1988:303-363.

8. Pollock ML, Wilmore JH. *Exercise in Health and Disease, Evaluation and Prescription for Prevention and Rehabilitation*. 2nd ed. Philadelphia: W.B. Saunders; 1990:1-750.

9. DeBusk RF, Blomquist CG, Kouchoukos NT, et al. Identification and treatment of low-risk patients after acute myocardial infarction and coronary-artery bypass graft surgery. *N Engl J Med*. 1986;314:161-166.

10. DeBusk RF. American College of Physicians Position Paper. Evaluation of patients after recent acute myocardial infarction. *Ann Intern Med*. 1989;110:485-488.

11. Jette M, Landry F, Blumchen G. Cardiac rehabilitation in the Federal Republic of Germany: Klinik Roderbirken. *J Cardiopulm Rehabil*. 1988;9:341-349.

12. Sheps DS. *The Management of Post-Myocardial Infarction Patients*. New York: McGraw & Hill; 1987:71-85.

13. DeBusk RF, Haskell WL, Miller NH, et al. Medically directed at-home rehabilitation soon after uncomplicated acute myocardial infarction: a new model for patient care. *Am J Cardiol*. 1985;55:1524-1528.

14. Gettman LR, Pollock ML, Ward A. Adherence to unsupervised exercise. *Physician & Sportsmed*. 1983;11:56-66.

15. King AC, Taylor CV, Haskell WL, DeBusk RF. Strategies for increasing early adherence to long-term maintenance of home-based exer-cise training in healthy middle-aged men and women. *Am J Cardiol*. 1988;61:628-632.

16. Greenland P, Chu JS. Efficacy of cardiac rehabilitation services with emphasis on patients after myocardial infarction. *Ann Intern Med*. 1988;109:650-663.

17. Wenger NK. Rehabilitation for coronary patients. Is ECG monitoring necessary? *Cardiovasc Persp*. 1988;2(4):4-6.

18. Haskell WL. Cardiovascular complications during exercise training of cardiac patients. *Circulation*. 1978;57:920-925.

19. Van Camp SP, Peterson RA. Cardiovascular complications of outpatient cardiac rehabilitation programs. *JAMA*. 1986;256:1160-1163.

20. Hellerstein HK, Franklin BA. Exercise testing and prescription. In: NK Wenger, HK Hellerstein, eds. *Rehabilitation of the Coronary Patient, 2nd edition*. New York: John Wiley & Sons; 1984:197-284.

21. DeBusk RF, Valdes R, Houston N, Haskell W. Cardiovascular responses to dynamic and static effort soon after myocardial infarction, application to occupational assessments. *Circulation*. 1978;58:368-375.

22. Kelemen MH, Stewart KJ, Gillilan RE, et al. Current weight training in cardiac patients. *J Am Coll Cardiol*. 1986;7:38-42.

23. Ghilarducci LE, Holly RG, Amsterdam EA. Effect of high resistance training in coronary artery disease. *Am J Cardiol*. 1989;64:866-870.

24. Wenger NK. Rehabilitation of the patient with acute myocardial infarction during hospitalization: early ambulation and patient education. In: ML Pollock, DH Schmidt, eds. *Heart Disease and Rehabilitation*. 2nd ed. New York: John Wiley & Sons; 1986:405-421.

25. Block A, Maeder JP, Haissly JC, Felix J, Blackburn H. Early mobilization after myocardial infarction. A controlled study. *Am J Cardiol*. 1974;34:152-157.

26. Clausen JP. Circulatory adjustments to dynamic exercise and physical training in normal subjects and in patients with coronary artery disease. In: EH Sonnenblick, M. Lesch, eds. *Exercise and the Heart*. New York: Grune & Stratton; 1977:39-75.

27. Thompson PD. The benefits and risks of exercise training in patients with chronic coronary artery disease. *JAMA*. 1988;259:1537-1540.

28. Jorgensen CR, Gobel FL, Taylor HL, Wang Y. Myocardial blood flow and oxygen consump-

tion during exercise. *Ann NY Acad Sci.* 1977; 301:213-223.

29. Foster C, Pollock ML, Anholm JD, et al. Work capacity in left ventricular function during rehabilitation after myocardial revascularization surgery. *Circulation.* 1984;69:748-755.

30. Detry J-MR, Rousseau M, Vandenbroucke G, Kusumi F, Brasseur LA, Bruce RA. Increased arteriovenous oxygen difference after physical training in coronary heart disease. *Circulation.* 1971;64:109-118.

31. Ehsani AA, Biello DR, Schultz J, Sobel BE, Holloszy JO. Improvement of left ventricular contractile function in patients with coronary artery disease. *Circulation.* 1986;74:350-388.

32. Leon AS. Comparative cardiovascular adaptation to exercise in animals and man and its relevance to coronary artery disease. In: CM Bloor, ed. *Comparative Pathophysiology of Circulatory Disturbances.* New York: Plenum Publishing; 1972:173-174.

33. Scheuer J. Effects of physical training on myocardial vascularity and perfusion. *Circulation.* 1982;66:491-495.

34. Kramsch DM, Aspen AJ, Abramowitz BM. Reduction of coronary atherosclerosis by moderate conditioning exercise in monkeys on an atherogenic diet. *N Engl J Med.* 1981;305: 1483-1488.

35. Bloor CM, White FC, Sanders TM. Effects of exercise on collateral development in myocardial ischemia in pigs. *J Appl Physiol Respir Environ Exerc Physiol.* 1984;56:656-665.

36. Rose G, Prineas R, Rhell JRA. Myocardial infarction and the intrinsic calibre of the coronary arteries. *Br Med J.* 1986;29:548-552.

37. Ferguson RG, Petticlerc R, Choquette G, et al. Effect of physical training on treadmill exercise capacity, collateral circulation and progression of coronary disease. *Am J Cardiol.* 1974; 34:764-769.

38. Connor JF, LaCamera F Jr, Swanick EJ, et al. Effects of exercise on coronary collateralization —angiographic studies of six patients in a supervised exercise program. *Med Sci Sports Exerc.* 1976;8:145-151.

39. Sim DN, Neill WA. Investigation of the physiological basis for increased exercise threshold for angina pectoris after physical conditioning. *J Clin Invest.* 1974;51:763-770.

40. Redwood DR, Rosing DR, Epstein SE. Circulatory and sympomatic effects of physical train-ing in patients with coronary heart disease and angina pectoris. *N Engl J Med.* 1972;286: 959-965.

41. Ehsani AA, Health GH, Hagberg JM, Sobel BE, Holloszy JO. Effects of 12 months of intense exercise training on ischemic ST segment depression in patients with coronary artery disease. *Circulation.* 1981;164:1116-1124.

42. Froelicher V, Jensen D, Genter F, et al. A randomized trial of exercise training in patients with coronary heart disease. *JAMA.* 1984;252: 1291-1297.

43. Sebrechts CP, Klein, JL, Ahnve S, Froelicher VF, Ashburn WL. Myocardial perfusion changes following 1 year of exercise training assessed by thallium-201 circumferential count profiles. *Am Heart J.* 1986;112:1217-1226.

44. Myers J, Ahnve S, Froelicher V, et al. A randomized trial of the effects of 1 year of exercise training on computer-measured ST segment displacement in patients with coronary artery disease. *J Am Coll Cardiol.* 1984;4:1094-1102.

45. Leon AS. Exercise and risk of coronary heart disease. In: HM Eckert, AJ Montoye, eds. *Exercise and Health. American Academy of Physical Education Papers.* No. 17. Champaign, IL: Human Kinetics Publishers; 1984:14-31.

46. Garrow JS. Effects of exercise on obesity. *Acta Med Scand.* 1986;(Suppl 711):67-74.

47. Haskell WL. The influence of exercise training on plasma lipids and lipoproteins in health and disease. *Acta Med Scand.* 1986;711(Suppl): 25-38.

48. Hagberg JM, Seals DR. Exercise training and hypertension. *Acta Med Scand.* 1986;711(Suppl): 131-136.

49. Holloszy JO, Schultz J, Kusnierkiewicz J, Hagberg JM, Ehsani AA. Glucose tolerance and insulin resistance. *Acta Med Scand.* 1986; (Suppl 711):61-73.

50. Dishman RK. Medical psychology in exercise and sports. *Med Clin North Am.* 1985;69: 123-143.

51. Hughes JR. Psychological effects of habitual aerobic exercise. A critical review. In: A. Leon, ed. *Forum: Exercise and Health. Prev Med.* 1984;13:66-78.

52. Blumenthal J, Emery CF, Rejeski WJ. The effects of exercise and psychosocial functioning after myocardial infarction. *J Cardiopulm Rehabil.* 1988;8:183-193.

53. Stern MJH, Cleary P. The National Exercise

and Heart Disease Project: long-term psychological outcomes. *Arch Intern Med*. 1982;142: 1093-1097.

54. Powell KE, Thompson PD, Caspersen CJ, Kendrick JS. Physical activity and incidence of coronary heart disease. *Annu Rev Public Health*. 1987;8:253-287.

55. Paffenbarger RS, Hyde RT. Exercise in the prevention of coronary heart disease (1984). In: A. Leon, ed. *Forum: Exercise and Health. Prev Med*. 1984;13:3-22.

56. Leon AS. Leisure-time physical activity levels and risk of coronary heart disease and death. The Multiple Risk Factor Intervention Trial. *JAMA*. 1988;258:2388-2395.

57. Sobloski J, Kornizer M, Abramowicz M. Protection against ischemic heart disease in the Belgium Physical Fitness Study: physical fitness rather than physical activity? *Am J Epidemiol*. 1987;125:601-610.

58. Peters RK, Cady LD, Bischoff DP, Bernstein L, Pike MC. Physical fitness and subsequent myocardial infarction in healthy workers. *JAMA*. 1983;249:3052-3056.

59. Naughton J. *Exercise Testing. Physiological, Biomechanical and Clinical Principles*. Mount Kisco, NY: Futura Pub. Co.; 1988:191-212.

60. Rechnitzer P, Cunningham DA, Andrew GM, et al. Relation of exercise to recurrence rate of myocardial infarction in men. Ontario Exercise Heart Collaborative Study. *Am J Cardiol*. 1983;51:65-69.

61. Vermueulen A, Lie K, Durer D. Effects of cardiac rehabilitation after myocardial infarction: changes in coronary risk factors and long-term prognosis. *Am Heart J*. 1983;105:798-801.

62. Kallio V, Hamalainen H, Hakkila J, Luurila OJ. Reduction of sudden deaths by a multifactorial intervention programme after acute myocardial infarction. *Lancet*. 1979;2:1091-1094.

63. May GS, Eberlein KA, Furberg CD, Passamani ER, DeMets DL. Secondary prevention after myocardial infarction: a review of long-term trials. *Prog Cardiovasc Dis*. 1982;24:331-362.

64. Pollock ML. Benefits of exercise on mortality and physiological function. In: CF Kappagoda, PV Green, eds. *Long-Term Management of Patients after Myocardial Infarction*. Boston: Martinus Nijhoff; 1988:189-205.

65. Oldridge NB, Guyait GH, Fischer ME, Rimm AA. Cardiac rehabilitation after myocardial infarction. Combined experience of randomized clinical trials. *JAMA*. 1988;260:945-950.

66. O'Connor GT, Buring JE, Yusaf S, et al. An overview of randomized trials of rehabilitation with exercise after myocardial infarction. *Circulation*. 1989;80:2:234-244.

67. Hossack KF, Hartwig R. Cardiac arrest with supervised cardiac rehabilitation. *J Cardiac Rehabil*. 1982;2:402-408.

68. Fletcher GF, Cantwell JD. Ventricular fibrillation in a medically supervised cardiac exercise program. *JAMA*. 1977;23:2627-2629.

# The Efficacy of Risk Factor Intervention and Psychosocial Aspects of Cardiac Rehabilitation

Nancy Houston Miller, RN; C. Barr Taylor, MD;
Dennis M. Davidson, MD; Martha N. Hill, RN, PhD;
Davis S. Krantz, PhD

Cardiac rehabilitation programs enhance the psychosocial functioning of individuals suffering from coronary heart disease. In formal rehabilitation programs this enhancement of psychosocial functioning is accomplished through education and risk factor modification, through evaluation of psychological status, and interventions such as support groups, individual therapy, and the direct contact provided by other coronary patients and staffs. The focus of this report is to define what is presently known about the psychosocial aspects of rehabilitation and to clearly identify the effectiveness of interventions in enhancing psychosocial functioning. Divided into two sections, risk factor modification and general psychosocial problems, task force members have assessed the extent of the problem, the rationale for intervention, the effectiveness of interventions, and have provided recommendations for management of patients within formal rehabilitation programs.

## Risk Factor Modification

Secondary prevention of coronary heart disease (CHD) through risk factor modification is potentially an important beneficial strategy that complements both medical and surgical interventions in attempting to reduce the risk of further CHD events. However, the understanding of the benefits of secondary prevention through risk reduction is limited by the lack of controlled studies to assess the significance of intervention strategies. Thus, the effects of interventions must be inferred in part from primary prevention studies in patients without manifest CHD.[1,2] Recent evidence, however, suggests that modification of certain risk factors after a coronary event such as a myocardial infarction (MI) may have substantial impact on morbidity and mortality.[3-5]

The first section of this report describes what is known about secondary prevention through risk factor modification. This section will address smoking, blood cholesterol, body weight, hypertension, diabetes, stress, and adherence. The benefits of exercise training have been fully described in a previous report and therefore will not be addressed here.[5]

### Smoking Cessation

A summary report citing many of the important epidemiologic studies has shown substantial reductions in death rates due to CHD following the cessation of smoking.[6] Moreover, for those patients who quit smoking after MI, there is a reduced risk of reinfarction, sudden cardiac death, and total mortality, compared to those who continue to smoke.[7,8] For instance, Sparrow found an 18.8% mortality rate six years after MI in men who

Note. This article is from the *Journal of Cardiopulmonary Rehabilitation*, 1990;10:198-209. Copyright 1990 by J.B. Lippincott Company. Adapted by permission.

The authors gratefully acknowledge Erika Sivarajan Froelicher, RN, PhD; Anne M. Dattilo, MS, RD; James Blumenthal, PhD; William P. Marley, PhD; William K. Wilkison; Martha Livingston, RN, MS, MBA; and other members of the 1989 and 1990 AACVPR board of directors for their help in reviewing the manuscript.

quit smoking, compared to a 30.4% mortality in those who maintained or resumed their smoking status after infarction.[7] The mechanism for this reduced risk is not known. Presumably smoking continues to contribute to the progression of atherosclerosis. Smokers have increased levels of plasma fibrinogen[9] and an increased frequency of silent ischemia[10] and arrhythmias.[11] One or several of these mechanisms may be plausible explanations of the etiology.

The rates of smoking in the general population have dropped during the past 20 years.[12] In the United States, however, it is unclear as to whether there has been a significant decline in the percentage of patients smoking at the time of an MI. In a recent American study, Taylor reported 46% of patients smoking within the six months prior to infarction.[13] Because smoking is a risk factor for CHD, smoking rates probably always will exceed those rates for the age-adjusted general population, which is now approximately 30%. It can be anticipated, therefore, that greater than 30% of the population with established CHD will be smoking at the time of an event.

There is a consensus that smoking cessation and maintenance of cessation are complicated phenomena involving both psychological and physiological dependence.[14,15] Nicotine is a highly addictive drug, with both stimulating and tranquilizing effects depending on the dosage. Smokers learn to regulate nicotine levels both to avoid withdrawal and to achieve the psychological effects.[11] In addition to the pharmacologic effects, the psychological effects of smoking are related to many aspects of a person's life. After quitting, smoking relapse occurs because a patient is unable to cope with urges, withdrawal symptoms, or the consequences of stopping.

A variety of techniques have been developed to help patients quit smoking. The effectiveness of interventions varies, depending on the population and nature of the intervention. The following conclusions, however, can be drawn from several studies: (1) most smokers quit on their own; (2) interventions combining multiple components are more successful than those relying on a single component; (3) nicotine gum combined with behavioral counseling may increase cessation rates; (4) for individuals successful at quitting, the greatest problem is relapse, preparation for which must be included in the overall cessation plan; and (5) health care professionals can be powerful facilitators of smoking behavior change.[14,16,17]

Among the cardiac population, cessation rates of 50% or more have been reported by a number of groups employing secondary prevention services, and situations in which the physician and medical team are committed to smoking cessation efforts.[18,19] According to Mulcahy,[20] smoking cessation rates of 46% in 1961-63 increased to 58% in 1973-75 and to as high as 70% in 1978-81. He attributes the change to greater effort employed by cardiac rehabilitation staff in implementing smoking cessation.[20] In a review of several studies, a 0-35% difference between treatment and control patients was found at six months or longer post-MI.[21,22] The most effective results occurred when close follow-up advice was provided to patients. A recent controlled study of post-MI patients using nurses to provide a relapse prevention behavioral intervention, revealed a biochemically confirmed cessation rate of 71% in an intervention group compared to 45% in a usual care group, a statistically significant difference.[23]

In summary, the evidence for the need for smokers with CHD to quit comes largely from observational epidemiologic studies. Such studies indicate that patients who continue to smoke post-MI have a higher morbidity and mortality compared to those who stop smoking. Stopping smoking after a cardiac event is the single most important lifestyle change to reduce subsequent morbidity and mortality. Multi-component strategies that start early in recovery and incorporate the use of behavioral techniques, strong physician advice, and the use of pharmacologic agents appear to achieve greater long-term cessation rates.

## Blood Cholesterol

An elevated serum total cholesterol level is firmly established as one of the major risk factors in the development of coronary artery disease and in the progression of disease among those with established atherosclerosis.[24,25] It is well-established that CHD morbidity and mortality is directly related to low-density lipoprotein (LDL) levels and inversely proportional to high-density lipoprotein (HDL) levels.[26] New data also indicate that HDL-C is a powerful risk factor, independent of elevated LDL.[27] Moreover, studies of patients with established CHD indicate that lowering serum cholesterol reduces risk of subsequent CHD events.[28] Recent investigations indicate that aggressive lipid management in this population may actually slow the progression of CHD.[29,30]

Dietary interventions have been undertaken to reduce blood cholesterol as part of primary prevention efforts. In the Oslo Heart Study, 1,232 healthy men were involved in a five-year randomized trial to show whether lowering serum lipids and cessation of smoking could reduce the incidence of CHD. In this study dietary manipulation (<30% total fat, <10% saturated fat, and <300 mg cholesterol) was associated with a 13% decrease in plasma cholesterol after five years. Dietary intervention in conjunction with smoking resulted in a 47% decrease in fatal and nonfatal MIs.[31]

Although there have been no clinical trials of dietary interventions aimed at secondary prevention, one study showed delayed progression in CHD-patients consuming a low-fat, low-cholesterol diet. In the Leiden Intervention Trial, patients followed a vegetarian diet for two years. Atherosclerotic lesion growth was prevented in 18 of the 39 patients while lesions progressed in 21 of 39; progression was more common in those whose total cholesterol remained above the median throughout the trial.[32]

The Coronary Drug Project, a trial of 8,341 men who had suffered an MI, was designed to lower patients' total cholesterol with one of five agents: estrogen in one of two doses, clofibrate, dextrothyroxine, nicotinic acid, and a placebo. During the trial both the estrogen and dextrothyroxine treatments were discontinued due to excessive cardiovascular events. In patients receiving nicotinic acid, however, a significant reduction in nonfatal MIs was noted that was still apparent 15 years after the trial.[3] In a 10-year follow-up study of coronary artery bypass surgery patients, baseline and ten-year serum total cholesterol levels were correlated directly with new atherosclerotic lesions. High LDL and low HDL levels were the best predictors of disease progression.[33] Blakenhorn[30] studied 162 men following coronary artery bypass surgery. Treatment included a diet low in fat, saturated fat and cholesterol and a combination of colestipol and nicotinic acid, or a placebo for a period of two years. Atherosclerotic progression was significantly less in those patients taking colestipol and niacin versus placebo. Regression occurred in 16.2% of patients treated with colestipol-niacin versus 2.4% of placebo patients (P<0.002). The improved global arteriographic changes were noted in men at all levels of baseline total cholesterol (range 185-350 mg/dl).[30]

A change in eating habits is the first recommendation for treatment of patients with elevated blood cholesterol. The National Cholesterol Education Program has recommended that patients with cardiovascular disease and with an LDL cholesterol >130 mg/dl begin a progressive two-stage plan to change dietary habits. The first stage is the Step-One diet to include reduction of total fat to <30% of total daily calories, comprised of saturated fat <10%, polyunsaturated fat <10%, and remaining fat from monounsaturated fatty acids; cholesterol intake is reduced to <300 mg/day. The American Heart Association indicates that cholesterol should decline about 10-15% with the Step-One diet. If additional cholesterol lowering is needed, patients advance to the Step-Two diet, which further limits saturated fat to <7% and cholesterol to 200 mg/day. If after six months of dietary intervention LDL cholesterol values remain above 130 mg/dl, these patients should be treated with lipid-lowering medications.[34]

A reduction in CHD events is noted as LDL levels fall. Many patients, however, will be unable to achieve recommended LDL cholesterol levels through a change in eating habits and may require drug therapy. Cholestyramine, nocotinic acid, and gemfibrozil have been found to be effective in clinical trials, as well as the new class of HMG CoA reductase inhibitors such as Lovastatin.[35-37] Health care professionals working in rehabilitation programs have an opportunity to provide education about specific medications, monitor side effects, tailor behavioral strategies to enhance patients' compliance to these drugs, and provide periodic reinforcement for patients' efforts. Through prompt identification of patients' problems with diet intervention and drug therapy and referral to physicians, this long-term follow-up of patients, especially those in the early stages of recovery, may enhance outcome.

In summary, the risks of hyperlipidemia and the effectiveness of diet and pharmacologic therapy of same, have been documented in patients under close supervision after coronary angioplasty, MI, and coronary artery bypass surgery, in addition to patients with documented CHD, without an event. Intervention with diet and drugs will continue to require considerable attention to behavior change principles and monitoring of adherence.

## Obesity/Weight Reduction

Obesity is a state of altered body composition with an increase in the proportion of body fat. The majority of epidemiologic studies relating weight to increased disease risk uses body mass index

(BMI), which adjusts weight for height (BMI = body weight in kg/height in meters, squared), whereas others define obesity in terms of percent body fat or the distribution of fat in certain defined areas that may be associated with greater morbidity and mortality. The National Obesity Consensus Conference in 1985 considered obesity to be 20% above ideal body weight for adults. This corresponds to a BMI above 26.4 for men and 25.8 for women.[38] The NIH Obesity Consensus Statement estimates that there are 34 million obese adult Americans.[38] Since obesity contributes to other risk factors and may independently increase CHD risk, at least 20% of patients with known CHD are likely to be obese.

Observational studies link obesity to hypertension, hypercholesterolemia, and diabetes.[39,40] Blood pressure, for example, varies directly with levels of obesity and can be lowered by weight reduction. Framingham data suggest that among males, a 10% reduction in body weight/BMI lowers cholesterol by 11 mg/dl, systolic blood pressure by 5 mm Hg, and blood glucose by 2 mg/dl.[41,42] The evidence associating obesity with CHD independent of other risk factors is less well-established. Some studies have shown obesity to be an independent risk factor for CHD[43] while others have not.[44] However, the NIH Consensus Development Conference concluded that the evidence of continuously increasing health risk with increasing relative weight was persuasive and that a level of 20% or more above desirable body weight is sufficiently associated with an increased risk to health to justify clinical intervention.

Losing weight and maintaining weight loss are difficult for most people. However, a recent review of 21 studies in the last five years reported a mean weight loss between 7 and 9 kg immediately after treatment.[45] The weight loss was related to the length of the program rather than the technique used. It appears to be more difficult for people to maintain weight loss than to lose it in a weight loss program. Many patients gain weight soon after a treatment program ends. However, eight recent studies reported a 75% maintenance of post treatment weight losses at one-year follow-up.[45] Regular exercise has been associated with better maintenance of weight loss.

Weight changes have been used as outcome measures in a number of post-MI exercise and multifactorial risk reduction intervention trials in cardiac patients. A few of these trials have found a significantly greater weight loss in the treatment group versus control group,[46,47] while one trial reported a reduction in body fat.[48] In all of these trials, however, the mean weight loss was less than 3 kg. Other weight loss studies have found no changes in weight.[49-51] A major problem with these studies in cardiac patients has been the lack of indication as to how many subjects were overweight and how much weight patients needed or wanted to lose.

Some patients with massive obesity and cardiovascular disease may have cardiac complications, such as congestive heart failure or hypertension, which may be significantly improved by massive weight loss. In such cases a very low-calorie diet may be considered. However, such low-calorie diets have been associated with various medical complications and must be used with great care in this population.

In summary, weight loss appears to be important in the cardiac population, especially in the obese group. It can be assumed that the principles for moderate weight loss developed for the normal population are equally useful in the cardiac population. In general, a reduction in fat intake to <30% of calories and increased exercise have only a modest effect on lowering weight. Therefore, cardiac patients needing to lose weight usually require some additional caloric restriction to facilitate weight reduction. Also, patients with massive obesity and cardiac disease may benefit from a more strict low-calorie weight loss program.

## Hypertension

Approximately 58 million Americans have hypertension (systolic blood pressure greater than or equal to 140 mg Hg and/or diastolic blood pressure greater than or equal to 90 mg Hg) or are taking antihypertensive medications.[52] Hypertension increases with age in all groups, although it is most prevalent in blacks and those with a personal and family history of high blood pressure, are older than 50 years, obese, diabetic, or have a heavy alcohol intake. The incidence of cardiovascular disease (particularly stroke) and mortality increases with systolic and diastolic blood pressure, more for men than women.[53] Furthermore, the risks from elevated blood pressure are independent from those of other known cardiovascular risk factors. The majority of the morbidity and mortality associated with hypertension is experienced by the 70% of hypertensives who have diastolic blood pressure in the 90-104 mmHg range ("mild" hypertension).

The effectiveness of antihypertensive drugs in lowering arterial blood pressure and reducing complications, such as stroke, congestive heart failure, and renal failure, is well established. Nonpharmacologic or hygienic approaches to blood pressure control, especially weight reduction, alcohol moderation, and sodium restriction, have been shown to lower blood pressure and to enhance the effectiveness of pharmacologic therapy.[54]

Following an MI, a substantial decrease in blood pressure may indicate a reduction in myocardial function. Conversely, those who remain hypertensive after the event are at greater risk for recurrent CHD events or mortality when compared to normotensive patients.[55] Evidence also indicates that treatment of hypertension is beneficial in patients who already have suffered an MI. The Hypertension Detection and Follow-up study, for example, showed a 20% reduction in mortality in patients assigned to the treatment group following infarction.[56] Patients with diastolic blood pressure greater than 95 mmHg often will also benefit from medical therapy. However, because diuretics and beta blockers may adversely affect blood lipid levels, the patient's risk profile and possible adverse effects of therapy should be considered before recommendations for drug therapy are provided.[57]

Health education programs using a combination of strategies such as simplification of regimen, social support, and self-monitoring, have been shown to be beneficial in improving adherence to blood pressure regimens, particularly for patients who need support to initiate or continue self-management.[58-62] Cardiac rehabilitation programs provide an opportunity for continued monitoring of blood pressure, ongoing surveillance of medication adherence, general education by health care professionals, and continued reinforcement of patients' efforts. Such surveillance by health care professionals may improve patient adherence and long-term blood pressure reduction and reduce mortality due to stroke and hypertension-related morbidity.[63] Because patients have different goals or standards for self-management and vary in how much help and attention they want and need to manage their condition effectively,[64] strategies need to be tailored to each individual.

In summary, treatment of hypertension is important in secondary prevention of CHD. Investigation of the interrelationships of cardiovascular risk factors, risk reduction strategies, and pathophysiologic changes, optimal blood pressure levels and physiologic changes, as well as the benefit of treatment of mild hypertension, are important areas for future research. Through education and counseling strategies, health care professionals can play an important role in helping to improve patient compliance.

## Diabetes

Diabetes mellitus is found in approximately 11 million people in the United States today, with 5 million people not having been diagnosed.[65] Diabetes also is 50% more common in females than males.[65] Although diabetes is associated with many problems, such as neuropathy, peripheral vascular disease, and retinopathy, CHD is the most common cause of death in diabetic adults. Moreover, the mortality rate for diabetic women from CHD is as great as the rate for nondiabetic men of the same age.[66]

Although diabetes, especially Type II or adult onset, is associated with a familial genetic predisposition, obesity appears to be the greatest precipitating factor for its development.[67] Glucose intolerance is an important direct effect of obesity, which is associated with hypertriglyceridemia, hypertension, and elevated LDL cholesterol.

Due to high mortality rates in this population, efforts to control risk factors in those with already established CHD becomes critical. Therefore, health care professionals in rehabilitation should be aware of the important components in the management of this disease which include: (1) caloric restriction of diet for those with obesity; (2) a diet high in complex carbohydrates (55%-60%), and low in total fat (no greater than 30%-35% of calories/fat and high in mono saturated fats); (3) control of plasma glucose levels with the use of insulin or oral hypoglycemic agents; and (4) moderate daily endurance type exercise, which may promote a plasma glucose lowering effect.[68] Special attention to the management of other risk factors, including hypertension and hyperlipidemia, also becomes important in this population.

## Stress, Type A Behavior and Hostility

A recent investigation implicated mental stress as a trigger of myocardial ischemia in CHD patients.[69] Moreover, research on psychosocial factors has been stimulated by the fact that many new cases of CHD are not predicted by the standard biologic risk factors.[70] This research has examined social indicators (e.g., socioeconomic status), characteristics of the environment (e.g., occupational stress and social support), and psychological factors such as Type A behavior and hostility. Comprehensive reviews of the literature on psychosocial variables can be found in Krantz et al., Manuck, Kaplan and Matthews, Matthews and Haynes, and Ostfeld and Eaker.[71-74]

The most extensively researched psychosocial variable relevant to CHD is the Type A behavior pattern (TABP). First identified by cardiologists Friedman and Rosenman,[75] TABP is characterized by excessive competitive drive, impatience, hostility, and vigorous speech characteristics. In the 1960s and 1970s, numerous studies examined the relationship of Type A behavior to CHD. Since that time their measurement instruments have been refined. Beginning with the Western Collaborative Group Study (WCGS), results were almost uniformly positive in supporting an association between TABP and CHD in both men and women that were comparable to, and independent of, the effects of the standard risk factors. However, in the last six years, other major studies, comprising mainly high risk groups, have failed to find a relation between TABP and coronary disease.[73] At least one study reported that Type A post-infarction patients survived longer post-MI than their Type B counterparts.[76]

Components of Type A behavior related to hostility or anger appear to be most strongly related to CHD. This conclusion is supported by studies re-analyzing components of the Structured Interviews used to assess TABP.[77,78] These studies have found that ''potential-for-hostility,'' defined as a predisposition to respond to frustration with reactions of anger, irritation, contempt, etc., was significantly associated with the future occurrence of CHD, even among sample groups who had not shown positive relationships between ''global'' TABP and coronary disease.[79,80]

The Cook-Medley Hostility Scale,[81] a self-report measure of cynical mistrust of others, also has been shown in several studies to be related to the incidence of CHD events as well as to the extent of coronary atherosclerosis.[82-84] However, two recent studies have failed to find that the Cook-Medley hostility questionnaire was predictive of CHD.[85] However, the preponderance of evidence, using multiple methodologies, suggests that aspects of hostility and anger are toxic elements of TABP, whereas other TABP elements (e.g., competitive-

ness, time urgency) are of lesser importance. These results may account for some of the inconsistencies in the literature on global TABP.[86]

Several intervention strategies have been successful in modifying Type A behavior. One, the Recurrent Coronary Prevention project, is a clinical trial designed to determine whether TABP modification using a cognitive social learning approach reduced recurrence of CHD in post-infarction patients.[87] Another large study involving 299 healthy Army staff, found that a combination of exercise and a cognitive behavioral intervention significantly reduced hostility as determined by the Structured Type A interview.[88] Roskies et al.[89] found that after a 10-week intervention, a stress management group showed greater changes in Type A behavior and components derived from the Structured Interview (SI) than an aerobic conditioning or weight-lift exercise group. Taken together, such studies indicate that it is possible not only to change global Type A but the hostility component of Type A. However, the long-term effects of such interventions remain uncertain. Also, standard measures of hostility and/or TABP need to be developed.

In summary, the role of TABP in its association with CHD is inconclusive with both positive and negative findings. Recent evidence suggests that hostility or anger may be the most important cardiovascular risk factor of Type A, but the data are still inconclusive. Further study is needed to determine if behavioral approaches to modification of TABP can reduce hostility in patients with established CHD and what the long-term effects of those interventions are.

## Adherence

Participation in cardiac rehabilitation programs may have some effect on adherence to medical regimens, although this issue has not been investigated in controlled trials. Two aspects of adherence may be affected by rehabilitation programs: (1) adherence to general aspects of treatment such as medication use; and (2) adherence to cardiovascular risk reduction behaviors. Regarding the former, there is evidence that ''health education'' in general can improve adherence to medical regimens. In a meta-analysis of adherence to education regimens among people with chronic illness, the average effect size for 70 published studies was 0.37, suggesting a significant beneficial effect of patient education on adherence.[90] To the extent that a cardiac rehabilitation program focuses on adherence, a similar effect could be anticipated.

There is less research on the effects of cardiac rehabilitation programs on adherence to risk-reduction behaviors. Several programs have reported high adherence rates to exercise for participants in cardiac rehabilitation programs. Oldridge and Jones[91] reported that adherence with a short program of three months' duration may exceed 80%, but adherence falls to 45-60% at 12 months and 30-55% at 48 months. Oldridge also has reported that including spouses in an exercise program increased compliance to 67-90%. The Stanford Cardiac Rehabilitation Program has reported exercise adherence rates of 89% and 84% for patients exercising 3-11 weeks post-infarction in home-based and group programs.[92] Between 11 and 26 weeks, these figures dropped to 72% and 71%, respectively.[92] The extent to which the results of Oldridge and Jones and the Stanford Cardiac Rehabilitation Program can be extended to non-research populations and settings is not known. Moreover, further work is needed to determine the effects of rehabilitation programs on adherence to weight loss, diet, medication use, and symptom response.

**Summary (Risk Factors)**

Few studies have evaluated the effectiveness of rehabilitation efforts designed to modify cardiovascular risk factors. The majority of studies have suffered from methodological problems such as small sample size and inadequate controls. Moreover, the interventions often have been very general, based on educational rather than behavioral approaches and without adequate evaluation designs.[2] However, at least one study has demonstrated that a post-MI multifactorial risk reduction program can be effective.[47] Other studies suggest that interventions for smoking and hyperlipidemia can reduce future CHD risks.[3-20] The demonstration that diet and medications can reduce hypercholesterolemia and progression of coronary atherosclerosis as documented by coronary angiography should encourage rehabilitative professionals to increase their efforts in these areas.

# General Psychosocial Issues and Intervention

In addition to risk factor management, psychological assessment and intervention are important for patients recovering from a CHD event. The main psychosocial factors that have been considered important to overall recovery include depression, anxiety, resumption of sexual activity, return to work, stress, and substance abuse. Problems of depression, anxiety, and social isolation, for example, have been shown to affect prognosis post-infarction.[93] Issues of resumption of sexual activity and return to work may significantly affect the patient's quality of life.[94,95] These issues not only relate to the patient but also to overall family functioning. The following sections will highlight the important aspects of managing these psychosocial issues and relate the effectiveness of cardiac rehabilitation efforts in this area.

**General Psychosocial Functioning (Well-Being)**

The general thought among health care professionals is that cardiac rehabilitation programs, most specifically exercise training, may improve psychosocial functioning. However, as noted in the AACVPR position paper on Exercise this has yet to be proven.[5] The number of studies is small, there is a lack of control subjects, and design problems are numerous. Even in the randomized, well-controlled studies[96-98] there is little evidence to support the role of exercise in improving psychological outcome.

What about other strategies for improving psychological functioning in the rehabilitation of coronary patients? The majority of other psychosocial interventions have been directed at improving the overall well-being of the patient. Interventions have included health education and counseling, individual and group psychotherapy, and stress management and relaxation. Nurses and other health care professionals have provided risk factor management and counseling about emotional adjustment in the inpatient and early outpatient phases of recovery after a coronary event.[98-100] In these randomized, controlled trials, improvements in psychosocial functioning (i.e., mood, distress, social support, knowledge of risk factors) were found to show statistical significance in the early (3-6 month) phases of recovery, a clinically important finding when measuring quality of life.[98-100] For example, assessing quality of life using the Sickness Impact Profile, Ott and co-workers,[98] found an improvement in psychosocial scales at three and six months after MI in those patients receiving an exercise program, or an exercise and counseling program versus a control group. A more recent controlled study by Burgess[100] showed that patients scored better on a distress scale and a scale of family support at three months post-MI, when they received a special teaching-counseling intervention provided by nurses. No significant improvements in occupational status have been noted in these studies.[98,100]

Other studies have used individual or group psychotherapy to effect psychosocial functioning in patients recovering from an MI. In a well-controlled study by Gruen,[101] a regimen of daily individual psychotherapy beginning in-hospital showed marked improvements in patient's depression, anxiety, and physical symptoms. At four months, patients receiving intervention had fewer episodes of cardiac problems and fewer hospitalization days.[101] Although the studies of group therapy demonstrate mixed results in relation to psychological improvement, some of these studies have shown significant improvements in facilitating recovery in various patient populations.

Finally, stress management and relaxation therapy programs also have been implemented to enhance psychosocial functioning in the coronary population. In a well-controlled study, Langosch[102] showed that patients who received in-hospital relaxation training and stress management performed better on psychological and vocational parameters at six months after discharge. In a more recent randomized study of stress, Frasure-Smith[103] showed that monitoring post-MI patients' stress levels by monthly telephone calls and using nurses to intervene with stress-reducing techniques (teaching, support, and consultation or referral) in the year after infarction produced a significant reduction in stress scores in the test group versus controls. Although re-hospitalizations and their duration did not differ, there were significantly fewer deaths in the monitored group.[103]

The studies noted suggest that health education and counseling, psychotherapy, and stress management show promising results in improving the quality of life in cardiovascular patients, especially those suffering an MI. In general, these studies have shown greatest improvements in the early phases of recovery. However, other studies addressing psychosocial outcomes have not shown statistically or clinically significant results. Methodologic problems, most notably small sample size and inadequate measurement tools, often have detracted from their impact.

## Depression/Anxiety

Depression and anxiety in the early days following an MI are almost universal.[104] However, depression and anxiety normally resolve spontaneously in the early course of recovery. Within three to four weeks after infarction or coronary artery bypass surgery, most patients are no longer depressed. Continued moderate to severe depression and anxiety occur in only 5-15% of patients according to two estimates based on small sample sizes.[105,106]

Severely depressed and anxious patients need intervention, for these co-morbidities may affect mortality.[107] Depression may be due to the life-threatening event, medications such as beta-blockers, or a pre-existing state. Anxiety may be present due to depression or other psychiatric problems, or may be chronic, associated with panic attacks. Sometimes anxiety and depression are related to the patient's uncertainty and lack of information about his condition.

Moderate to severe depression can be identified through simple screening tools.[108] Referral for therapy and identification of patients taking beta-blocking agents that may be causing depression are important tasks for rehabilitation staff. Many patients will recover with brief psychotherapy, but antidepressants may be indicated for severe depression. Exercise also may reduce depression in clinically depressed patients after MI.[109] However, the studies that have examined the effects of exercise on reducing anxiety and depression and improving mood or sense of well-being in nonpsychologically impaired populations are inadequate.[110]

Anxiety disorders also may occur in patients with CHD.[111] One type of anxiety disorder is called panic disorder because of the characteristic panic attacks (sudden episodes of fear accompanied by such symptoms as dyspnea, sweating, dizziness, palpitations, choking, fear of going crazy, or losing control).[111,112] Such patients should be referred for specialized treatment.

## Sexual Dysfunction

Sexual problems are not uncommon following an MI or coronary artery bypass surgery. The frequency of sexual intercourse may decrease by 24-75% in middle-aged men following an MI.[113] The most commonly cited reasons for the dysfunction are symptoms of fatigue and angina, psychological fears that an event such as an MI has damaged the patient (resulting in depression or lowered self-esteem), and medications such as beta-blocking agents and diuretics, which cause sexual impairment.[94] It is unclear as to whether cardiac rehabilitation programs, specifically exercise, have a positive impact on sexual function, including interest and desire. However, it is known that failure of health care professionals to discuss this topic may contribute to sexual dysfunction in the post-MI population.[114] Lack of detailed instructions and failure to refer people for appropriate counseling at the time of an event may lead to depression and lack of resumption.[115] Therefore, adequate counseling in the form of education and referral to psychologists, physicians, and sexual therapists for problems such as impotence and loss of libido are clearly within the scope of cardiac rehabilitation efforts.

## Return to Work

Although not all patients choose to go back to work following an event such as an MI or CABG bypass surgery, returning to normal activities, including work, is important to many patients recovering from acute cardiac events. The proportion of patients returning to work after an MI ranges from 49% to 93%.[116-118] Physical, psychosocial, demographic, and clinical characteristics all influence resumption of work after such an event. Because these nonmedical factors[117,119] so strongly influence return to work, it may be difficult to show that exercise training through cardiac rehabilitation programs influences an earlier return. However, exercise training usually increases functional capacity, which for some patients may serve to enhance their effectiveness upon return.

Two issues deserve more attention in the area of returning to work and cardiac rehabilitation. Enhancing patients' perceptions about their health status and influencing their attitudes about returning to work through appropriate information about safety, risks, and prognosis may improve the likelihood that they will return to work. Perceived health status was correlated with return to work in MI and CABG patients independent of actual health status.[117,120] Alleviating misconceptions about occupational tasks, providing vocational counseling, and giving explicit advice about prognosis also may help to enhance patients' attitudes.

Health care professionals in rehabilitation are in a unique position to facilitate a safe, early return to work and optimal social functioning. Early exercise testing is routine for patients recovering from an MI. Recommendations about return to normal activities, including work, can be based on exercise test results. For example, a randomized clinical trial in post-MI patients demonstrated that patients who received a treadmill test and explicit instructions about the results, prognosis, and timing of return, actually returned to work at a median of 51 days compared to 75 days in patients receiving usual care.[121] Rehabilitation personnel often are involved in conducting treadmill testing or providing the counseling thereafter during which such information can be given and reinforced. Such efforts may not only help to influence the timing of return but may also make patients feel more comfortable about coping with work-related stressors.

## Alcohol/Substance Abuse

Much attention has been focused in recent years on the relationship between alcohol and HDL cholesterol. Specifically, even a small consumption of alcohol causes a rise in the HDL cholesterol subfraction which is thought to exert a protective CHD effect.[122] The protective effect, however, appears to be dose-dependent, and heavy consumption of alcohol is associated with adverse lipid and lipoprotein levels and increased CHD risk.[123]

Although alcohol in moderate doses may exert a positive effect on lipids, there is also a positive correlation between alcohol and hypertension. Significant increases in both systolic and diastolic blood pressure have been noted in patients consuming more than three drinks per day.[124]

In patients suffering CHD, heavy alcohol intake may impede recovery. Severe alcohol abuse may interfere with compliance to changing risk factors and may produce atrial and ventricular arrhythmias and impaired ventricular functioning.[125,126]

Approximately 8-10% of adults consider themselves to be alcoholic. Patients who are given firm, unambiguous instructions about the importance of treatment are more likely, with family support, to follow through with recommended advice for treatment.[127] Rehabilitation personnel have the ability to adequately assess alcohol abuse through such instruments as the Michigan Alcohol Screening Instrument[128] and the CAGE questionnaire[129] and to make an adequate referral when appropriate. Such effort is needed to enhance the psychosocial and physical recovery of these patients.

Cocaine, another powerful substance, is used in epidemic proportions in our country today. In 1974, approximately 5.4 million people were using cocaine. The prevalence of cocaine use sharply increased to 22.2 million in 1986, and it is estimated that from 5 to 6 million Americans are using it regularly.[130]

The effects of cocaine on the heart have been documented mainly from observational case studies over the past few years. Cardiac complications have included myocarditis, dilated cardiomyopathy, cardiac arrhythmias, aortic rupture, pulmonary edema, and MI and death.[131,132] Noted since 1982, an MI may occur in patients with normal or diseased coronary arteries after the use of cocaine, although the exact pathophysiologic mechanism when this occurs is unknown.[133] It also has been observed that continued cocaine use may be particularly hazardous to these patients because recurrent myocardial ischemic syndromes and MI have occurred with repeated use.

Rehabilitation personnel should ask information about cocaine and other drug use in screening patients. All patients using cocaine should be told emphatically that they must stop and be provided with a referral for treatment.

### Summary (General Psychosocial Problems)

Various psychosocial factors are important to the overall recovery of patients who suffer CHD events. Cardiac rehabilitation programs provide an opportunity for identification of patients having severe psychosocial problems. In this environment, these patients can be adequately screened, offered available programs, or referred for further long-term management.

It remains unclear as to whether interventions in the cardiac rehabilitation setting improve psychosocial outcome. The use of groups for education and counseling as part of cardiac rehabilitation have been demonstrated to improve quality of life in a few well-designed randomized trials.[82-84] These studies have produced only modest improvements in psychosocial functioning.

Clearly (as with risk factor modification) additional well-controlled studies and confirmatory studies of those showing promising results are needed to prove the benefit of cardiac rehabilitation. In the past, general approaches to study in this area often have yielded vague results. More specific interventions targeting specific psychosocial outcomes are likely to lead to better results. Until such studies are conducted, rehabilitation professionals need to continue to adequately screen and refer patients when appropriate to improve psychosocial outcomes.

## References

1. Hartley LH, Foreyt JP, Alderman MH, et al. Task Force 6: secondary prevention of coronary artery disease. *Circulation.* 1987; 76(Suppl):I-168-I-173.

2. Godin G. The effectiveness of interventions in modifying behavioral risk factors of individuals with coronary heart disease. *J Cardiopulm Rehabil.* 1989;9:223-236.

3. Canner PL, Berge KG, Wenger KN, et al. Fifteen year mortality in Coronary Drug Project patients: long-term benefit with niacin. *J Am Coll Cardiol.* 1986;8:1245-1255.

4. Aberg A, Bergstrand R, Johansson S, et al. Cessation of smoking after myocardial infarction: effects on mortality after 20 years. *Br Heart J.* 1983;49:416-422.

5. Leon AS, Certo C, Comoss P, et al. Scientific evidence of the value of cardiac rehabilitation services with emphasis on patients following myocardial infarction. Section 1. Exercise conditioning component. *J Cardiopulm Rehabil.* 1990;10:79-87.

6. The health consequences of smoking: cardiovascular disease. A report of the Surgeon General. Rockville, MD: U.S. Department of Health and Human Services. PHHS (84-50204, 1983).

7. Sparrow D, Dawber TR, Colton T. The influence of cigarette smoking on prognosis after a first myocardial infarction. *J Chronic Dis.* 1978;31:425-432.

8. Rosenberg L, Kaufman DW, Helmrich SP, Shapiro S. The risk of myocardial infarction after quitting smoking in men under 55 years of age. *N Engl J Med.* 1985;313:1511-1514.

9. Meade TW, Imeson J, Stirling Y. Effects of changes in smoking and other characteristics on clotting factors and the risk of ischaemic heart disease. *Lancet.* 1987;986-988.

10. Barry J, Mead K, Nabel EG, et al. Effect of smoking on the activity of ischemic heart disease. *JAMA.* 1989;261:398-402.

11. Benowitz NL. Pharmacologic aspects of cigarette smoking and nicotine addiction. *N Engl J Med*. 1988;319:1318-1329.

12. Schwartz JL. *Review and evaluation of Smoking Cessation Methods: the United States and Canada 1978-1985*. Washington, DC: Division of Cancer Prevention and Control, National Cancer Institute; 1987:1-6. NIH Publication No. 87-2940.

13. Taylor CB, Houston-Miller N, Haskell WL, DeBusk RF. Smoking cessation after acute myocardial infarction: the effects of exercise training. *Addict Behav*. 1988;13:331-335.

14. Taylor CB, Houston-Miller N. Smoking cessation in patients with cardiovascular disease. *Qual Life Cardiovasc Care*. 1989;5:19-35.

15. Lichtenstein E. The smoking problem: a behavioral perspective. *J Consult Clin Psychol*. 1982;50:804-819.

16. Green HL, Goldberg RJ, Ockene JK. Cigarette smoking: the physician's role in cessation and maintenance. *J Gen Intern Med*. 1988;3:81-87.

17. Schwartz JL. *Review and Evaluation of Smoking Cessation Methods: The United States and Canada 1978-1985*. Washington, DC: Division of Cancer Prevention and Control, National Cancer Institute; 1987:15-132. NIH Publication No. 87-2940.

18. Burling TA, Singleton GE, Bigelow GE, Baile WF, Gottlieb SH. Smoking following myocardial infarction: a critical review of the literature. *Health Psychol*. 1984;3:83-96.

19. Burt A, Thornby P, Illingworth D, White P, Shaw TRD, Turner R. Stopping smoking after myocardial infarction. *Lancet*. 1974; 1:304-306.

20. Mulcahy R. Influence of cigarette smoking on morbidity and mortality after myocardial infarction. *Br Heart J*. 1983;49:410-415.

21. Schwartz JL. *Review and Evaluation of Smoking Cessation methods: The United States and Canada 1978-1985*. Washington, DC: Division of Cancer Prevention and Control, National Cancer Institute; 1987:53-58. NIH Publication No. 87-2940.

22. Sivarajan ES, Newton KM, Almes MJ, Kempf TM, Mansfield LW, Bruce RA. Limited effects of outpatient teaching and counseling after myocardial infarction: a controlled study. *Heart Lung*. 1983;12:65-73.

23. Taylor CB, Miller NH, Killen JD, DeBusk RF. Smoking cessation after acute myocardial infarction: effects of a nurse-managed intervention. *Ann Intern Med*. 1990;113:118-123.

24. Dawber TR. *The Framingham Study*. Cambridge, MA: Harvard University Press; 1980.

25. Schlant RC, Forman S, Stamler J, et al. The natural history of coronary heart disease: prognostic factors after recovery from myocardial infarction in 2,789 men. The 5-year findings of the Coronary Drug Project. *Circulation*. 1982;66:401-414.

26. Kannel WB. Contributions of the Framingham Study to the conquest of coronary artery disease. *Am J Cardiol*. 1988;62:1109-1112.

27. Kannel WB. HDL cholesterol as a predictor of coronary heart disease and mortality: results from Framingham. In: *Symposium on Dyslipoproteinemia and Coronary Heart Disease: The Significance of HDL Cholesterol*. 1986:5.

28. Castelli WP, Garrison RJ, Wilson RWF, Abbott RD, Kalousdian S, Kannel WB. Incidence of coronary heart disease and lipoprotein cholesterol levels: the Framingham study. *JAMA*. 1986;256:2835-2838.

29. Brown GB, Lin TJ, Schaefer SM, et al. Niacin or lovastatin, combined with colestipol, regress coronary atherosclerosis and prevent clinical events in men with elevated apoliprotein B. *Circulation*. 1989;80:II-266.

30. Blankenhorn DH, Nessim SA, Johnson RL, et al. Beneficial effects of combined colestipol-niacin therapy on coronary atherosclerosis and coronary venous bypass grafts. *JAMA*. 1987;257:3233-3240.

31. Hjerman L, Holme I, Velve Brye K, Leren P. Effect of diet and smoking intervention on the incidence of coronary heart disease. *Lancet*. 1981;1303-1310.

32. Arntzenius AC, Kromhout D, Barth JD, et al. Diet, lipoproteins, and the progression of coronary atherosclerosis. The Leiden Intervention Trial. *N Engl J Med*. 1985;312:805-811.

33. Campeau L, Enjalbert M, Lesperance J, et al. The relation of risk factors to the development of atherosclerosis in the saphenous vein bypass grafts and the progression of disease in the native circulation: a study 10 years after aortocoronary bypass surgery. *N Engl J Med*. 1984;311:1329-1332.

34. National Cholesterol Education Program. Report of the National Cholesterol Education Program Expert Panel on Detection, Evaluation, and Treatment of High Blood Cholesterol in Adults. *Arch Intern Med*. 1988; 148:38-69.

35. The Lipid Research Clinic Coronary Primary Prevention Trial Results. I. Reduction in incidence of coronary heart disease. *JAMA*. 1984;251:351-364.

36. The Lipid Research Clinic Primary Prevention Trial Results. II. The relationship of reduction in incidence of coronary heart disease to cholesterol lowering. JAMA. 1984;251:365-374.

37. Frick MH, Elo O, Haapa K. Helsinki Heart Study. *N Engl J Med*. 1987;317:1237-1245.

38. National Obesity Consensus Conference. *Ann Intern Med*. 1985;100(Suppl):888-900.

39. Miller HW. *Plan and Operation of the Health and Nutrition Examination Survey, United States, 1971-1973: A Description of the National Health and Nutrition Examination Survey of a Probability Sample of the U.S. Population 1-74 Years of Age*. Hyattsville, MD: National Center for Health Statistics; 1985. DHEW Publication No. (PHS) 79-1310. Vital and Health Statistics: Series 1, No. 10a.

40. Keys A, Aravanis C, Blackburn H, et al. Coronary heart disease: overweight and obesity as risk factors. *Ann Intern Med*. 1972;77:15-27.

41. Ashley FW, Kannel WB. Relation of weight change to changes in atherogenic traits: the Framingham study. *J Chronic Dis*. 1974; 27:103-114.

42. Kannel WB, Gordon T. Obesity and some physiological and medical concomitants: the Framingham study. In: GA Bray, ed. *Obesity in America*; 1979:125-162. Washington, DC: U.S. Government Printing Office. NIH Publication No. 79-359.

43. Hubert HB, Feinleib M, McNamara PM, Castelli WP. Obesity as an independent risk factor for cardiovascular disease: a 26-year follow-up of participants in the Framingham Heart Study. *Circulation*. 1983;67:968-977.

44. Garrison RJ, Feinleib, Castelli WP, McNamara PM. Cigarette smoking as a confounder of the relationship between relative weight and long-term mortality: the Framingham Heart Study. *JAMA*. 1983;249:2199-2203.

45. Brownell KD, Jeffery RW. Improving long-term weight loss: pushing the limits of treatment. *Behav Ther*. 1987;18:353-374.

46. Wilhelmsen L, Sanne H, Elmfeld D, Grimby G, Tibblin G, Wdel H. A controlled trial of physical training after myocardial infarction. *Prev Med*. 1975;4:491-508.

47. Kallio V, Hamalainen H, Hakkila J, Luurila OJ. Reduction in sudden deaths by a multifactorial intervention programme after acute myocardial infarction. *Lancet*. 1979;2:1091-1094.

48. Oberman A, Cleary P, Larosa JC, Hellerstein HK, Naughton J. Changes in risk factors among participants in a long-term exercise rehabilitation program. *Adv Cardiol*. 1982; 31:168-175.

49. Marra S, Paolillo V, Spadaccini F, Angelino PF. Long-term follow-up after a controlled randomized post-myocardial infarction rehabilitation programme: effects on morbidity and mortality. *Eur Heart J*. 1985;6:656-663.

50. Carson P, Phillips R, Lloyd M, et al. Exercise after myocardial infarction: a controlled trial. *J R Coll Physicians London*. 1982;26:147-151.

51. Vermeulen A, Lie KI, Burrer D. Effects of cardiac rehabilitation after myocardial infarction: changes in coronary risk factors and long-term prognosis. *Am Heart J*. 1983; 105:798-801.

52. Hypertension prevalence and the status of awareness, treatment, and control in the United States: final report of the Subcommittee oon Definition and Prevalence of the 1984 Joint National Committee. *Hypertension*. 1985;7:457-468.

53. Lerner DJ, Kannel WD. Patterns of coronary heart disease morbidity and mortality: a 26 year follow-up of the Framingham population. *Am Heart J*. 1986;111:383-390.

54. The 1988 Joint National Committee on Detection, Evaluation, and Treatment of High Blood Pressure. *Arch Intern Med*. 1988; 148:1023-1038.

55. Kannel WB, Sorlie P, Castelli WP, McGee D. Blood pressure and survival after myocardial infarction: the Framingham study. *Am J. Cardiol*. 1980;45:326-330.

56. Langford HG, Stamler J, Wasserthiel-Smoller S, Prineas RJ. All cause mortality in the Hypertension Detection and Follow-up Program: findings for the whole cohort and for persons with less severe hypertension with and without other traits related to the risk of mortality. *Prog Cardiovasc Dis*. 1986;29:29-54.

57. Weinberger MH. Antihypertensive therapy and lipids: paradoxical influences on cardio-

vascular disease risk. *Am J Med.* 1986; 80:64-70.

58. Levine DM, Green LW, Deeds SG, et al. Health education for hypertensive patients. *JAMA.* 1979;241:1700-1703.

59. Levine DM, Green LW. State of the art in research and evaluation. *Bull NY Acad Med.* 1985;61:135-143.

60. Hypertension Detection and Follow-up Program Cooperative Group: five year findings of the Hypertension Detection and Follow-up Program. I. Reduction in mortality of persons with high blood pressure, including mild hypertension. *JAMA.* 1979;242:2562-2571.

61. Multiple Risk Factor Intervention Trial Research Group: Multiple Risk Factor Intervention Trial: risk factor changes and mortality results. *JAMA.* 1982;248:1465-1477.

62. Haynes RB. A critical review of the determinants of patient compliance with therapeutic regimens. In: DL Sackett, RB Haynes, eds. *Compliance with Therapeutic Regimens.* Baltimore, MD: Johns Hopkins University Press; 1976:26-39.

63. Working Group on Health Education and High Blood Pressure Control, National High Blood Pressure Education Program. *The Physician's Guide: Improving Adherence Among Hypertensive Patients.* Bethesda, MD: U.S. Department of Health and Human Services, National Heart, Lung and Blood Institute; March 1987.

64. Hill MN. Strategies for patient education. *Clinical and Experimental Hypertension—Theory and Practice.* 1989;A11(5 and 6): 1187-1201.

65. American Diabetes Association. *Diabetes Facts and Figures.* Alexandria, VA: American Diabetes Association; 1986.

66. Barrett-Connor E, Orchard T. Diabetes and heart disease. In: NI Harris, RF Hamman, eds. *Diabetes in America.* Bethesda, MD: National Institutes of Health; 1986. NIH Publication No. 85-1468.

67. West KM. Epidemiology of diabetes and its vascular lesions. New York: Elsevier; 1978:1.

68. Leon, A. Patients with diabetes mellitus. In: BA Franklin, ed. *Exercise in Modern Medicine.* Baltimore, MD: Williams and Wilkins; 1989:118-145.

69. Rozanski A, Bairey CN, Krantz DS, et al. Mental stress and the induction of silent myocardial ischemia in patients with coronary

artery disease. *N Engl J Med.* 1988; 318:118-145.

70. Jenkins CD. Psychosocial and behavioral factors. In: N Kaplan, J Stamler, eds. *Prevention of Coronary Heart Disease.* Philadelphia, PA: Saunders Publications; 1983:98-112.

71. Krantz DS, Contrada RJ, Hill DR, Friedler E. Environmental stress and biobehavioral antecedents of coronary heart disease. *J Consult Clin Psychol.* 1988;56:333-341.

72. Manuck SB, Kaplan JR, Matthews KA. Behavioral antecedents of coronary heart disease and atherosclerosis. *Arteriosclerosis.* 1986;6:1-14.

73. Matthews KA, Haynes SG. Type A behavior pattern and coronary disease risk: update and critical evaluation. *Am J Epidemiol.* 1986;123:923-960.

74. Ostfeld A, Eaker E, eds. Measuring psychosocial variables in epidemiologic studies of cardiovascular disease. Bethesda, MD: National Institutes of Health; 1985. NIH Publication No. 85-2270.

75. Friedman M, Rosenman RH. Association of specific overt behavior pattern with blood and cardiovascular findings: blood cholesterol level, blood clotting time, incidence of arcus senilis, and clinical coronary artery disease. *JAMA.* 1959;169:1286-1296.

76. Ragland DR, Brand RJ. Type A behavior and mortality from coronary heart disease. *N Engl J Med.* 1988;318:65-69.

77. Matthews KA, Glass DC, Rosenman RH, Bortner RW. Competitive drive, pattern A and coronary heart disease: a further analysis of some data from the western collaborative group study. *J Chronic Dis.* 1977;30:489-498.

78. Hecker MHL, Chesney MA, Black GW, Frautschi N. Coronary-prone behaviors in the Western Collaborative Group Study. *Psychosom Med.* 1988;2:153-164.

79. Dembroski RM, MacDougall JM, Costa PT, Grandits GA. Components of hostility as predictors of sudden death and myocardial infarction in the Multiple Risk Factor Intervention Trial. *Psychosom Med.* (In press).

80. MacDougall JM, Dembroski TM, Dimsdale JE, Hackett TP. Components of Type A, hostility, and anger. In: Further relationships to angiographic findings. *Health Psychol.* 1985;4:137-152.

81. Cook WW, Medley DM. Proposed hostility

and pharisaic virtue scales for the MMPI. *J Appl Psychol*. 1954;38:414-418.

82. Williams RB, Haney TL, Lee KL, Kang V, Blumenthal JA, Whalen RE: Type A behavior, hostility, and coronary atherosclerosis. *Psychosom Med*. 1980;42:529-538.

83. Shekelle RB, Gale M, Ostfeld A, Paul O. Hostility, risk of coronary heart disease and mortality. *Psychosom Med*. 1983;45:109-114.

84. Barefoot JC, Dahlstrom WC, Williams RB. Hostility, CHD incidence, and total mortality: a 25-year follow-up study of 255 physicians. *Psychosom Med*. 1983;45:59-63.

85. McCranie EW, Watkins LO, Brandsma JM, Sisson BD. Hostility, coronary heart disease (CHD) incidence, and total mortality: lack of association in a 25-year follow-up study of 478 physicians. *J Behav Med*. 1986; 9:119-126.

86. Krantz DS, Manuck SB. Acute psychophysiologic reactivity and risk of cardiovascular disease: a review and methodologic critique. *Psychol Bull*. 1984;96:435-464.

87. Friedman M, Thoresen CE, Gill JJ, et al. Alteration of Type A behavior and its effect on cardiac recurrences in post myocardial infarction patients: summary results of the Recurrent Coronary Prevention Project. *Am Heart J*. 1986;112:653-665.

88. Schaeffer MA, Krantz DS, Weiss SM, et al. Effects of occupational based behavioral counseling and exercise interventions on Type A components and cardiovascular reactivity. *J Cardiopulm Rehabil*. 1988; 10:371-377.

89. Roskies E, Seraganian P, Oseasohn R, et al. The Montreal Type A Intervention Project: major findings. Health Psychol. 1986; 5:45-69.

90. Mullen PD, Green LW, Persinger G. Clinical trials of patient education for chronic conditions: a comparative meta-analysis of intervention types. *Prev Med*. 1985; 14:753-781.

91. Oldridge NB, Jones NL. Preventive use of exercise rehabilitation after myocardial infarction. *Acta Med Scand*. 1986;711(Suppl): 123-129.

92. Miller NH, Haskell WL, Berra K, DeBusk RF. Home versus group exercise training for increasing functional capacity after myocardial infarction. *Circulation*. 1984; 70:645-649.

93. Mumford E, Schlesinger H, Glass G. The effects of psychological intervention on recovery from surgery and heart attacks: an analysis of the literature. *Am J Public Health*. 1982;72:141-151.

94. Kolman PB. Sexual dysfunction in the postmyocardial infarction patient. *J Card Rehabil*. 1984;4:334-340.

95. Fitzgerald ST. Occupational outcomes after treatment for coronary heart disease: a review of the literature. *Cardiovasc Nurs*. 1989;25:1-4.

96. Stern MJ, Cleary P. The National Exercise and Heart Disease Project: long-term psychological outcome. *Arch Intern Med*. 1982; 142:1093-1097.

97. Erdman RA, Duivenvoorden HJ. Psychologic evaluation of a cardiac rehabilitation program: a randomized clinical trial in patients with myocardial infarction. *J Card Rehabil*. 1983;3:696-704.

98. Ott CR, Sivarajan ES, Newton KM, et al. A controlled randomized study of early cardiac rehabilitation: The Sickness Impact Profile as an assessment tool. *Heart Lung*. 1983;12:162-170.

99. Pozen MW, Stechmiller JA, Harris W, Smith S, Fried DD, Voigt GC. A nurse rehabilitator's impact on patients with myocardial infarction. *Med Care*. 1977; 15:830-837.

100. Burgess AW, Lerner DJ, D'Agostino RB, Vokonas PS, Hartman CR, Gaccione P. A randomized control trial of cardiac rehabilitation. *Soc Sci Med*. 1987;24:359-370.

101. Gruen W. Effects of brief psychotherapy during the hospitalization period on the recovery process in heart attacks. *J Consult Clin Psychol*. 1975;43:223-232.

102. Langosch W, Seer P, Brodner G, Kallinke D, Kulick B, Heim F. Behavior therapy with coronary heart disease patients: results of a comparative study. *J Psychosom Res*. 1982;26:475-484.

103. Frasure-Smith N, Prince R. The Ischemic Heart Disease Life Stress Monitoring Program: impact on mortality. *Psychosom Med*. 1985;47:431-445.

104. Cassem NH, Hackett TP. Psychiatric consultation in a coronary care unit. *Ann Intern Med*. 1971;75:9.

105. Taylor CB, DeBusk RF, Davidson DM. Optimal methods for identifying depression following hospitalization for myocardial infarction. *J Chronic Dis*. 1981;34:127-133.

106. Hackett TP. Depression following myocardial infarction. *Psychomatics*. 1985; 26(Suppl):23-28.

107. Ruberman W, Weinblatt AB, Goldberg JD, Chaudbury BS. Psychosocial influences on mortality after myocardial infarction. *N Engl J Med*. 1984;311:552-559.

108. Beck AT, Weissman A, Lester D, Trexler L. The measurement of pessimism: The Hopelessness Scale. *J Consult Clin Psychol*. 1974; 42:861-865.

109. Taylor CB, Sallis J, Needle R. The relationship of exercise and physical activity to mental health. *Public Health Rep*. 1985; 100:195-202.

110. Hughes JR. Psychological effects of habitual aerobic exercise: a critical review. In: A Leon, ed. *Forum. Exercise and Health. Prev Med*. 1984;66-78.

111. Taylor CB, Arnow B. The nature and treatment of anxiety disorders. New York: The Free Press; 1985:313-314.

112. Taylor CB, Sheikh J, Agras WS, et al. Ambulatory heart rate changes in patients with panic attacks. *Am J Psychiatry*. 1986; 143:479-482.

113. Mann S, Yates JE, Raftery EB. The effects of myocardial infarction on sexual activity. *J Card Rehabil*. 1981;1:187-193.

114. Baggs J, Karch A: Sexual counseling of women with coronary heart disease. *Heart Lung*. 1987;16:154-158.

115. Papadopoulos C, Beaumont C, Shelley SI, Larrimore P. Myocardial infarction and sexual activity of the female patient. *Arch Intern Med*. 1983;143:1528-1530.

116. Cay EL, Vetter N, Philip A. Return to work after a heart attack. *J Psychosom Res*. 1973; 17:231-243.

117. Garrity TF. Vocational adjustment after first myocardial infarction: comparative assessment of several variables suggested in the literature. *Soc Sci Med*. 1973;7:705-717.

118. Nagle R, Gangola R, Picton-Robinson I. Factors influencing return to work after myocardial infarction. *Lancet*. 1971; 2:454-456.

119. Smith GR, O'Rouke DF. Return to work after myocardial infarction. *JAMA*. 1988; 259:1673-1677.

120. Gundle NJ, Reeves BR Jr, Tate S, Raft D, McLaurin LP. Psychosocial outcome after coronary artery surgery: a randomized clinical trial. *Am J Psychiatry*. 1980; 137:1591-1594.

121. Dennis C, Houston-Miller N, Schwartz RG, et al. Early return to work after uncomplicated myocardial infarction. Results of a randomized trial. *JAMA*. 1988;260:214-220.

122. Haskell WL, Camargo C Jr, Williams PT, et al. The effect of cessation and resumption of moderate alcohol intake on serum high-density-lipoprotein subfractions: a controlled study. *N Engl J Med*. 1984;310:805-810.

123. Lieber CS. To drink or not to drink? *N Engl J Med*. 1984;310:846-848.

124. Klatsky AL, Friedman GD, Sjegelaub AB, Gerard MJ. Alcohol consumption and blood pressure: Kaiser-Permanente multiphasic health examination data. *N Engl J Med*. 1977; 296:1194-1199.

125. Gould L, Gopolaswamy C, Yang D, et al. Effect of oral alcohol on left ventricular ejection fraction, volumes and segmental wall motion in normals and in patients with recent myocardial infarction. *Clin Cardiol*. 1985;8:576-582.

126. Davidson DM. Cardiovascular effects of alcohol. *West J Med*. 1989;151:430-439.

127. Pattison EM. The alcoholic patient: clinical approaches. *Psychosomatics*. 1986;27:762-770.

128. Selzer ML. The Michigan Alcoholism Screening Test: the quest for a new diagnostic instrument. *Am J Psychiatry*. 1971; 127:1653-1658.

129. Ewing JA. Detecting alcoholism: the CAGE questionnaire. *JAMA*. 1984;252:1905-1907.

130. Schnoll SH, Daghestani AM, Hansen TR. Cocaine dependence. *Resident and Staff Physician*. 1984;30(11):24-31.

131. Isner JM, Estes M, Thompson PD, et al. Acute cardiac events temporally related to cocaine abuse. *N Engl J Med*. 1986;315:1438-1441.

132. Virmani R, Robinowitz M, Smialek JE, Smyth DF. Cardiovascular effects of cocaine: an autopsy study of 40 patients. *Am Heart J*. 1988;2:1068-1076.

133. Smith HWB, Liberman HA, Brody SL, et al. Acute myocardial infarction temporally related to cocaine use. *Ann Intern Med*. 1987;107:13-18.

# *Index*

**A**

Alcohol
  relationship with cholesterol, 97
  relationship with hypertension, 97
Alcohol and substance abuse, 97-98
  impeding recovery from coronary heart disease, 97
  suggested efficacy measures for program, 31
Anatomy and physiology, discussed in cardiac rehabilitation programs, 23
Anger, relationship with coronary heart disease, 94
Angina
  daily log for, 68
  indicating increasing risk of, 48-49
  and participation in exercise programs, 12
Anxiety disorders, 96
Arrhythmias
  daily log for, 68
  indicating increasing risk of, 49

**B**

Behavior change
  goals for, 18
  programs for, for cardiac patients, 18-20
Beta-blocking medication, causing depression, 96

**C**

Cardiac arrest. *See also* Cardiovascular complications
  incidence of, during exercise, 12-13, 39, 79, 83-84
  principles for management of, 61-62
Cardiac exercise therapy. *See* Cardiac rehabilitation
Cardiac patients. *See also* High-risk patients; Low-risk patients
  assessment of, 17-20
  behavior change programs for, 18-20
  benefits of exercise training for, 80-83
  characteristics of, 5
  contraindications to exercise testing of, 10, 12
  contraindications to exercise training for, 12
  ECG monitoring needed by, 5-6, 39, 55, 79
  educational services for, 20-23
  eligibility for cardiac rehabilitation services, 3
  high-risk patient profile, 38-40
  keeping records of, 44-46
  moving through phases of cardiac rehabilitation, 4
  risks of high-intensity training for, 13
  risk stratification for, 5, 78
  safety of cardiac exercise therapy for, 12-13, 83-84
  setting objectives for, 18
  weight training guidelines for, 11

Cardiac rehabilitation. *See also* Exercise training
  and adherence to medical regimens, 94-95
  American Association of Cardiovascular and Pulmonary Rehabilitation Guidelines for, 2
  assessing program effectiveness, 27-31
  behavior change as a goal of, 18
  benefits of, 80-83
  changes in, since 1970s, 2-3
  components of, 77-78
  defined, 3
  ECG monitoring during, 5-6, 39, 79
  educational services, 20-23
  effective exercises for, 10
  efficacy of risk factor intervention, 89-98
  emergency management in, 47-52
  estimated requirements for, 80
  evidence of the value of, 77-84
  facilities and equipment needed for, 53-56
  goals and objectives of, 4, 18, 77
  incidence of cardiovascular complications, 12-13, 39, 83-84
  phases of. *See* In-hospital programs; Outpatient convalescent programs; Outpatient maintenance programs; Maintenance programs
  process of, 3-4
  psychological intervention as part of, 23, 95, 96
  psychosocial issues, 95-98
  record-keeping guidelines, 43-46
  risk-factor counseling needed with, 5-6
  risk-stratification guidelines for, 5
  safety of, 12-13, 83-84
  spectrum of patients eligible for, 3
  technology to assist, 3
  weight training for, 10-11
Cardiac rehabilitation personnel, 33-38, 77-78
  availability of, 39-40
  competency standards for, 34-38
  educational standards for, 34-38
  emergency training recommended for, 48
  exercise specialist, 36
  health educator, 37
  medical director/supervising physician, 35
  mental health professional, 37
  minimal requirements, 35-36
  nutritionist, 36-37
  occupational therapist, 38
  pharmacist, 38
  physical therapist, 37-38

Cardiac rehabilitation personnel (continued)
  program director/coordinator, 35-36
  recommended additional personnel, 36-38
  registered nurse, 36
  responsibilities of, 34
  staff-to-patient ratio, 39-40
  training and certification for emergency management, 48
  utilization in supervision of exercise therapy, 40
  vocational rehabilitation counselor, 37
Cardiovascular complications
  during cardiac exercise therapy, 12-13, 79, 83-84
  interventions in response to, 49-50, 61-62
  recommendations to reduce, 13
  risk of, 38-40
  warning signs of, 48-49
Cardiovascular efficiency, improved by exercise training, 81
Cholesterol
  connection with coronary heart disease, 90-91
  diet and drug therapy to reduce, 90-91
  programs to reduce, 19, 90-91
  relationship with alcohol, 97
Cocaine, 97-98
  effects on the heart, 98
Coronary heart disease, possible protective effect of exercise training, 82-83
Coronary heart disease risk factors
  diabetes, 93
  discussed in cardiac rehabilitation programs, 22
  elevated serum cholesterol, 90-91
  hypertension, 92-93
  modification of, 89-95
  obesity, 91-92
  reduced by exercise training, 81-82
  smoking, 89-90
  stress, 93-94

D
Depression and anxiety, intervention needed for, 96
Diabetes
  link with coronary heart disease, 93
  link with obesity, 93
Diabetic program
  and expected outcomes, 20
  suggested efficacy measures for, 30

E
ECG monitoring
  cost of, 5, 6
  criteria for, 6, 79
  need for, 39, 55
  during Phase II, 5-6
  use questioned, 6, 79
Educational services, 20-23
  principles and resources for, 21-22
  program content for, 22-23
  teaching strategies, 20-21
  use of national standards recommended for, 21-22
Emergency cart checklist, 72-73
Emergency equipment, 38-39, 50-51

Emergency management, 47-52
  documentation for, 51-52, 59-74
  early warning signs of cardiovascular complications, 48-49
  emergency equipment needed for, 50-51
  interventions, 49-50
Equipment. See Facilities and equipment
Exercise specialist, 36
Exercise testing. See also Exercise training
  cardiac arrest associated with, 13
  contraindications to, 10, 12
  needed emergency equipment for, 51
  during outpatient convalescent programs (Phase II), 79
  during Phase III programs, 80
  predischarge tests, 10
  procedures for, 9-10
  purposes of, 10, 78, 79
Exercise therapy informed consent form, 71
Exercise therapy record form, 70
Exercise training. See also Cardiac rehabilitation
  benefits of, 80-83
  cardiac arrest associated with, 13
  contraindications to, 12
  couteracting effects of inactivity, 80
  effective exercises for, 10
  improving cardiovascular efficiency, 81
  improving functional capacity, 80-81
  improving psychological well-being, 82
  increasing myocardial vascularity, 81
  modifying Type A behavior, 94
  potential for preventing secondary coronary heart disease events, 82-83, 89-95
  and psychological well-being, 82, 95
  reducing risk factors for coronary heart disease, 81-82
  relationship with psychosocial functioning, 95
  safety of high-intensity training questioned, 13
  weight training guidelines for, 11

F
Facilities and equipment, 53-56
  for adult resuscitations, 59-60
  balancing cost effectiveness and patient needs, 56
  for high-risk patients, 55, 56
  for in-hospital programs, 53-54
  for low-risk patients, 54, 55
  for maintenance programs, 55-56
  for moderate-risk patients, 54-56
  for outpatient programs, 54-55
  proper use of, 56
Functional capacity, improved by exercise training, 80-81

G
Graded exercise testing. See Exercise testing

H
Health educator, 37
High intensity training, risks of, 13
High-risk patient profile, 38-40
High-risk patients. See also Cardiac patients
  advantages of supervised exercise for, 79
  characteristics of, 5

facilities and equipment needed for, 55, 56
greater needs of, 40
prognosis for, 78
Hostility, relationship with coronary heart disease, 94
Hypertension
    effectiveness of drug therapy for, 93
    monitoring provided by cardiac rehabilitation programs, 93
    relationship with alcohol, 97
    relationship with coronary heart disease, 92-93
    risks resulting from, 92-93
Hypertension management programs
    and expected outcomes, 19
    suggested efficacy measures for, 30

I

Inactivity, countered by exercise training, 80
Individualized exercise program
    and expected outcomes, 19
    suggested efficacy measures for, 28-29
In-hospital programs (Phase I), 3, 4, 78
    emergency management in, 50
    facilities and equipment needed for, 53-54
    purpose of, 4
    record keeping for, 44
    types of therapy in, 4

L

Lipid modification program
    and expected outcomes, 19
    reducing coronary heart disease risks, 90-91
    suggested efficacy measures for, 29-30
Low-risk patients. See also Cardiac patients
    characteristics of, 5
    facilities and equipment needed for, 54, 55
    group settings an advantage for, 78-79
    prospects for, 78
    weight training guidelines for, 11

M

Maintenance programs (Phase IV), 4, 78
    facilities and equipment needed for, 55-56
    record keeping for, 45-46
Medical director/supervising physician, 35
Medical education, provided by cardiac rehabilitation programs, 22
Medical intervention, documentation for, 69
Mental health professional, 37
Mock code documentation, 74
Moderate-risk patients. See also Cardiac patients
    characteristics of, 5
    facilities and equipment needed for, 54, 55-56
Myocardial vascularity, possibly increased by exercise training, 81

N

Nutritionist, 36-37

O

Obesity
    contributing to other risk factors, 92
    link with diabetes, 93
    and risk of coronary heart disease, 91-92

Occupational therapist, 38
Outpatient convalescent programs (Phase II), 4, 78
    cardiovascular complications during, 12-13, 38-39, 79
    ECG monitoring during, 5-6, 39-40, 55
    ECG monitoring questioned, 79
    emergency management in, 50
    exercise testing during, 79
    facilities and equipment for, 54-55, 78-79
    record keeping for, 44-45
    role of arm exercise in, 79
    safety of, 12-13, 83-84
Outpatient maintenance programs (Phase III), 4, 78
    cardiovascular complications during, 12-13, 38-39
    emergency management in, 50
    exercising testing during, 80
    facilities and equipment needed for, 54-55
    patient qualifications for, 79-80
    record keeping for, 44-45

P

Patient assessment, 17-20. See also Cardiac patients
Patient education program, suggested efficacy measures for, 28
Patient information records, 44-46
Pharmacist, 38
Phase I. See In-hospital programs
Phase II. See Outpatient convalescent programs
Phase III. See Outpatient maintenance programs
Phase IV. See Maintenance programs
Physical therapist, 37-38
Physician standing order, 63-67
Program director/coordinator, 35-36
Program evaluation, 27-31
    suggested efficacy measures for, 28-31
Psychological and neuropsychological disorders therapy program and expected outcomes, 20
    suggested efficacy measures for, 31
Psychological well-being, and exercise programs, 82, 95
Psychosocial factors, and recovery from coronary heart disease events, 95-98
Psychosocial functioning
    alcohol and substance abuse, 97-98
    and cardiac rehabilitation programs, 82, 89
    depression and anxiety, 96
    positive effects of intervention on, 95-96
    relationship with exercise, 95
    return to work, 97
    sexual dysfunction, 96-97
    stress management, 96
Psychosocial intervention
    as part of cardiac rehabilitation programs, 23
    providers of, 95, 96

R

Registered nurse, 36
Return to work
    nonmedical influences on, 97
    role of cardiac rehabilitation programs, 97
Return-to-work programs
    and expected outcomes, 20
    suggested efficacy measures for, 31

Risk, symptoms of increase in, 48-49
Risk factor counseling, 5-6
Risk stratification guidelines, 5
Risk stratification tools, 78

S

Sexual dysfunction, 96-97
Signs and symptoms, discussed in cardiac rehabilitation
    programs, 22-23
Smoking
  aids to quitting, 90
  physiological effects of, 89-90
  psychological effects of, 90
Smoking abuse, 19
Smoking cessation
  effect on coronary heart disease risk, 89-90
Smoking cessation programs
  success rates for, 90
  suggested efficacy measures for, 29

Stress, 19, 93-94
    relationship with coronary heart disease, 94
Stress management, 96

T

Type A behavior pattern
    modified by exercise, 94
    relationship with coronary heart disease, 94

V

Vocational programs, as part of cardiac rehabilitation
    programs, 23
Vocational rehabilitation counselor, 37

W

Weight reduction programs, 91-92
  and expected outcomes, 19
  suggested efficacy measures for, 30
Weight training
  for cardiac exercise therapy, 10-11
  guidelines for, 11

# *About the AACVPR*

## Statement of Purpose

Recognizing that cardiovascular and pulmonary rehabilitation is a multidisciplinary field, the American Association of Cardiovascular and Pulmonary Rehabilitation (AACVPR) is dedicated to the improvement of clinical practice, promotion of scientific inquiry, and advancement of education for the benefit of the health-care professional and the public.

## Objectives

The AACVPR strives to

- provide professional education through sponsorship and/or promotion of educatinal conferences, scientific meetings, and publications;
- provide a forum for information exchange through a resource center that proactively communicates with health-care professionals to effect delivery of quality health-care services;
- encourage, coordinate, and/or sponsor research that will enhance understandings of rehabilitation impact on disease processes, the health and personal welfare of patients, and the social health-care support systems;
- promote throughout the public sector understandings as to the nature of rehabilitation and increase awareness of the related health-care services available across the nation;
- cooperate and/or collaborate with other organizations having interests similar to those of the Association;
- provide ways and means to enhance career development for Association members.

## Membership Benefits

- Receive the *Journal of Cardiopulmonary Rehabilitation* monthly, keeping you updated on current research and information in the field of rehabilitation.
- Be part of a national network of professionals dedicated to the advancement of cardiovascular and pulmonary rehabilitation.
- Receive a quarterly newsletter containing information about practical issues.
- Have the opportunity to attend regional seminars and the AACVPR Annual Meeting.
- Be included in and have access to the national membership directory and national program directory.
- Be a part of a great networking system and have access to nationwide job opportunities.
- Receive up-to-date information on federal and state guidelines, reimbursement for rehabilitation services, and other issues of concern to professionals in the field.
- Have the opportunity to publish articles in the *Journal of Cardiopulmonary Rehabilitation* and present original research at the Annual Meeting.

We invite you to meet the challenge and become involved in the AACVPR. Decide to join this dynamic organization today. Fill out the membership application included in this book and send it to the AACVPR. The professional growth that you will experience by becoming a member of this Association will benefit you for years to come. We look forward to your future support and contributions.

# American Association of Cardiovascular and Pulmonary Rehabilitation

## MEMBERSHIP APPLICATION

Name _____  Male ☐  Female ☐  ___/___/___
                                                      Birthdate

Mailing address _____
          Office or clinic

          _____
          Street

          _____
          City                    State        Zip/postal code
                                                ( )
          _____
          Country                              Telephone

---

## CURRENT PROGRAM INVOLVEMENT (Check all that apply)

Job title: _____

☐ Cardiovascular rehabilitation   ☐ Pulmonary rehabilitation   Other (specify): _____
  ☐ Inpatient                       ☐ Inpatient
  ☐ Outpatient                      ☐ Outpatient                _____

---

## MEMBERSHIP CATEGORIES

**Select and complete only one category. Requirements are listed on the back of this application.**

### MEMBER

| ☐ **Physician** | ☐ **Scientist** | ☐ **Allied health** | ☐ **Educator** | ☐ **Nurse** |
|---|---|---|---|---|
| ☐ Cardiology<br>☐ Pulmonary<br>☐ Internal medicine<br>☐ Family/general practice<br>☐ Other | •Degree(s): _____<br><br>•Principle field of education:<br>_____<br><br>•Certification/licensure: | •Degree(s): _____<br><br>•Principle field of education:<br>_____<br><br>•Certification/licensure: | •Degree(s): _____<br><br>•Principle field of education:<br>_____<br><br>•Certification/licensure: | •Degree(s): _____<br><br>•Certification/licensure:<br>_____ |
| _____<br>$95.00 per year | $95.00 per year | $95.00 per year | $95.00 per year | $95.00 per year |

| ☐ **STUDENT MEMBER** | ☐ **ASSOCIATE MEMBER** |
|---|---|
| Institution: _____<br>Major: _____<br>Full-time credit load at your institution: _____<br>Number of credits you are currently taking: _____<br>Year degree expected: _____<br>                    month        year<br>$50.00 per year | Primary occupation: _____<br>Institution: _____<br>Major area(s) of interest: _____<br><br>$95.00 per year |

Mail application with check or money order in
U.S. currency to:   **AACVPR**
                    7611 Elmwood Avenue, Suite 201
                    Middleton, WI 53562
                    608-831-6989

**I certify that the above information is correct, and I agree to abide by the Code of Ethics and Professional Conduct of the American Association of Cardiovascular and Pulmonary Rehabilitation.**

_____        _____
Signature                Date

**Where did you hear about the AACVPR?**

EB    T    M    AM    BD    NM    RM    _____

_____

*Membership in the AACVPR is on a calendar-year basis (January 1–December 31).*

# Code of Ethical and Professional Conduct

## A. Objectives

This code is designed to aid the Fellows and Members of the Association, individually and collectively, to maintain a high level of ethical and professional conduct. The code may be considered a standard by which a Fellow or Member may determine the propriety of his or her conduct and relationship with colleagues, members of allied professions, the public, and all persons with whom a professional relationship has been established. These should be concordant with the principal purpose of the Association, which is the improvement of clinical practice, promotion of scientific inquiry, and advancement of education for the benefit of health-care professionals and the public in the multidisciplinary field of cardiovascular and pulmonary rehabilitation.

Fellows and Members should strive continuously to improve their knowledge and skills and to make available to their colleagues and to the public the benefits of their professional attainments.

Fellows and Members should maintain high professional and scientific standards and should not voluntarily associate professionally with those who violate this principle.

The Association should safeguard the public and itself against Fellows or Members who are deficient in ethical conduct or professional competence.

## B. Maintenance of Good Standing in Regulated Professions

Any Fellow or Member required by law to be licensed, certified, or otherwise regulated by any government agency or professional association in order to practice his or her profession must remain in good standing before that agency or association as a condition of continued membership in the American Association of Cardiovascular and Pulmonary Rehabilitation. Any expulsion, suspension, probation, or other sanction imposed by such government or professional body on any Fellow or Member may be grounds for disciplinary action by the Association.

## C. Public Disclosure of Affiliation

Any Fellow or Member may make disclosure of affiliation with the Association in an appropriate professional context, including use in curriculum vitae, in biographical descriptions, or in another professional, dignified manner. Disclosure of affiliation may not be made in connection with any commercial venture without prior written authorization of the Association. A commercial venture is defined here to mean the sale of any goods, services, or other property for a valuable consideration with the exception of books, journal articles, or other professional publications. Requests for such authorization should be made in writing to the President or the Executive Director of the Association. Fellows may list their affiliation with the Association on professional or business cards, only by the use of the initials F.A.A.C.V.P.R.; members other than Fellows may not use this affiliation on business or professional cards. Disclosure in violation of these guidelines may be grounds for disciplinary action.

The use of the name of the American Association of Cardiovascular and Pulmonary Rehabilitation as a cosponsoring or cooperating organization for professional meetings, professional education programs, and the like must follow the guidelines of the Association for these specific designations.

## D. Discipline

Any Fellow or Member of the Association may be disciplined or expelled for conduct which, in the opinion of the Board of Directors, is derogatory to the dignity or inconsistent with the purposes of the Association. The expulsion of a Fellow or Member may be ordered upon the affirmative vote of two-thirds of the members of the Board of Directors present at a regular or special meeting and only after such Fellow or Member has been informed of the charges preferred and has been given an opportunity to refute such charges before the Board of Directors. Other disciplinary action such as reprimand, probation, or censure may be recommended by the Committee on Ethics and Professional Conduct and ordered following the affirmative vote of at least two-thirds of the members of the Board of Directors present at a regular or special meeting or by mail ballot, provided a quorum take action.

# Membership Requirements

## Member

Shall be any interested person of majority age who is a physician, medical scientist, allied health-care practitioner, or educator, and who in his or her professional endeavors, is regularly involved in some aspect of cardiovascular and/or pulmonary rehabilitation. Members have AACVPR voting privileges.

## Fellow

Shall be qualified as a Member; attended a minimum of two Annual Meetings; demonstrated high standards of professional development and a commitment to the goals and long-range activities of the Association; submitted evidence of outstanding performance in some aspect of cardiovascular or pulmonary rehabilitation over a period of at least five years relative to (a) clinical practice, (b) research, and/or (c) professional education in cardiovascular and pulmonary rehabilitation; received recommendations in writing by two Fellows of the Association; and received the approval of the Credentials Committee and the Board of Directors. Fellows have AACVPR voting privileges.

## Student Member

Shall be any interested college student currently carrying the equivalent of at least one half of an academic load for one year, as defined by the university or college the person is attending, and one who is studying in a medical or allied health curriculum.

## Associate Member

Shall be any person with an interest in cardiovascular and/or pulmonary rehabilitation, but not currently eligible for classification as a Member or Student Member. Dues are established by the Board of Directors and may be changed at its discretion. Associate Member privileges include a subscription to any AACVPR newsletter that may be published and placement on the Association mailing list.